PRAISE FOR

SILVER PLATTER GIRL

Trish Kinney's story is a classical story of survival behavior. The changes she created for herself are changes which lead to immune competence and the healing of one's life. For me, her experience can be summarized as being born again in the sense that it is the birth of something new in each of us which conquers death. Her acting experience, I am sure, was a help too. I am always telling people to act and behave as if they were the person they wanted to be. "Silver Platter Girl" shows that if you rehearse and practice who you want to be, it can happen, regardless of your past, when you realize you are a divine child and learn to love yourself.

—Dr. Bernie Siegel
  Author of NY Times bestseller, *Love, Medicine and Miracles*

Silver Platter Girl kept me thinking all day and all night. Ms. Kinney's blunt, raw truth of her survival of sexual abuse is like holding a mirror up to your own history and inspecting it directly - the good and the bad. Her willingness to share her trauma and her triumph had me truly analyzing my own life and relationships. She unwraps her trauma as her life story unfolds, in much the same way the trauma of abuse is layered on over time for many victims - it seeps into every aspect of your life - until you can't recognize your true self. Ms. Kinney introduces the reader to every aspect of the abuse that suffocates her to the point where she is faced with an illness that is a physical manifestation of her trauma.

Silver Platter Girl is about how each of us can find our inner resiliency and have a healing awakening, even if the catalyst is fighting and defeating a life-threatening illness. Thank you, Ms. Kinney, for baring your heart and soul for all survivors to know there is always hope for healing and finding themselves again.

—Diana McWilliams
  Executive Director, Santa Fe Rape Crisis &Trauma Treatment Center

In 25 years of practice in cancer care, Trish Kinney, more than any of my patients, has taught me the transforming power of the focused mind against this frightening disease. Her breast cancer, in terms of statistics and risk was a bad one. Her dogged determination to make her battle against cancer a success made more difference than all of our medical tools combined.

Trish taught me that health is a choice that a patient can make, even when facing dismal odds. Health, whether physical, mental or spiritual, begins as a choice to make negative circumstances work in your favor. This story tells of how innocence lost and the spiral of negative consequences can be turned around not only in spite of cancer but in some ways because of it. It shows how transformative mental imaging can create an extraordinary success not only against cancer and the side effects of treatment but also against childhood demons.

Like the home town of Phoenix from where she tells the story, her life after cancer has flowered from the ashes of her battle. I can only pray that others, both patients and non-patients alike, may catch the magic in her story and apply her principles of mental transformation in their own journey.

—**John K. Camoriano, MD**, FACP, Mayo Clinic Scottsdale Oncology

Accounts of pain are common. Honest accounts are rare. Writing honestly about it makes it hurt again. The only reason to revisit the emotional wounds endured by Trish Kinney is, in the telling, to be able to help someone else ... it is the same motivation that makes someone dash into a burning building or plunge into an icy river to save a stranger. If medals were given for books instead of reviews, *Silver Platter Girl* would merit a mix between a Purple Heart and the Congressional Medal of Honor.

—**FJ Camper,** author of *Mindbenders* and *The MK/Ultra Secret*

This is a no-holds-barred, courageous examination of how childhood abuse shapes a life and how honesty with oneself can lead to healing. It's also a very well-written terrific read.

—**Casey Dorman, Ph.D.**
Psychologist and author of *I, Carlos*

Trish Kinney is not only a survivor, but a victor in every area of her life. This book is a must read not only for survivors of sexual abuse, but for all who have the courage to face whatever life has to offer and continue that journey with optimism, hope and eventually the ability to love oneself.

—Claire R. Reeves, MA, C.C.D.C.
President/Founder Mothers Against Sexual Abuse, MASA
Author: Childhood – It Should Not Hurt

Trish is a psychological alchemist who has transformed her emotional and physical wounds from childhood, provoked by "indecent exposures," to a brave sacrifice of complete "exposure," healing herself as she weaves her tale. She has journeyed way beyond the intimate confines of the therapy room represented by the axiom "know thyself." In her book she has leaped into a whole different level of intimacy, something we all profess to want but don't have the relentless courage to pursue. *Trish has revealed herself.* Sharing the private details of her thoughts and experiences, she sparks a yearning in the reader to begin or continue their own journey of self discovery and find the gold found in one's own truth. As Trish expresses over and over again, "the truth will set you free."

Trish's book confronts addiction head on as we are transported deep into the oceanic crevices of her psyche. Suffering from the ultimate betrayal of childhood: a father's sexual exploitations and a powerless mother who could not protect her family, Trish loosens the boundary between how addiction to other people is not much different from other addictions. Trish's addiction to be desired reveals the unconscious attempt to contain her mass of undigested suffering and grief. Her story teaches us that there is no short cut from the necessary truth: *to avoid pain creates greater pain.* And then she got the ultimate wakeup call… her diagnosis of breast cancer in the form of a massive tumor. Trish's life had "grown" out of control, symbolizing the wounded feminine part of her.

As a dancer, already skilled in a relationship with her body, she used her diagnosis as a path to recovery. Being entrapped by her immense emotional and now physical suffering (and the survivor's guilt she held for her sisters suffering as well) brings to mind the wisdom of the late genius of modern dance, Martha Graham: the body doesn't lie. Trish teaches us the only true exit from our own suffering is *in the becoming a psychological being*. It is the active synthesis toward a more completed self, integrating all parts of the human experience: the intellectual, emotional, physical and spiritual life which initiates healing the painful split between the mind and heart. Trish takes another necessary truth in the healing journey: responsibility for one's own transgressions, knowing sometimes we need to go backwards in order to move forwards. She has a huge heart, big enough to forgive herself and her parents with just one non-negotiable demand: they must also quest for the truth and take responsibility for the hurt they caused.

Last but not least, Trish's story tells all of us we cannot do this journey alone. She has had three exceptional men in her life to support her and love her. This book is an ode to her two sons and husband equally brave in joining her on this journey.

—Joanna Dovalis, M.F.T. Ph.D
Co-Author, *Grieving, Therapy, Cinema* and *Kieslowski's Trois Couleurs: Blanc*

SILVER PLATTER GIRL

TRISH KINNEY

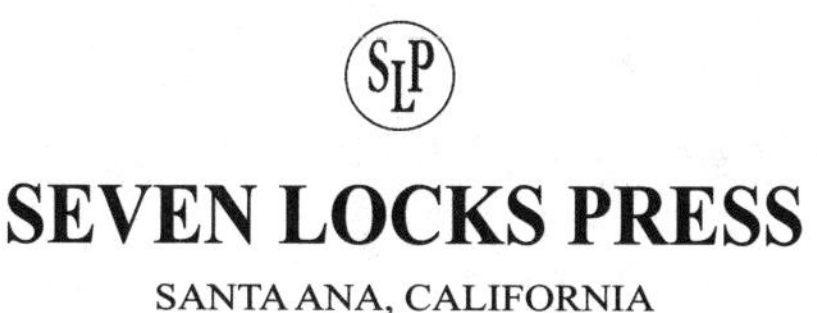

SEVEN LOCKS PRESS

SANTA ANA, CALIFORNIA

Seven Locks Press
P.O. Box 25689
Santa Ana, CA 92799
(800) 354-5348

Individual sales: This book is available through most bookstores or can be ordered directly from Seven Locks Press at the address above.

Quantity Sales: Special discounts are available on quantity purchases by corporations, associations and others. For details, contact the "Special Sales Department" at the publisher's address above.

Cover Image Peter Vander Stoep
Cancer Image Michael Smallwood

Design by Kira Fulks * www.kirafulks.com
Printed in the United States of America

Library of Congress Cataloging-in-Publication Data is available from the publisher

ISBN: 978-0-9822293-9-2   0-9822293-9-9

A C K N O W L E D G E M E N T

To my dear friend and partner, Kathy Leek, for her hard work, support, encouragement, inspiration, loyalty and trust.

To Joanne Osheel, for the invaluable gift of time to do this work and for knowing where I belong and making it possible for me to go there every day.

To Jim Riordan and Seven Locks Press for joining me out on the limb and believing in the power of the truth.

To Alicia, Estelle and Andria for their validation and for sharing their enormous talents with me and this project.

To Marvin Gaye. I did as you asked. You can rest now.

And to Jilly girl, the coyote dog, for staying by my side throughout the dark days of writing this story. We miss you.

OVERTURE

My first performing experience was as a very young child singing with my sister. My father encouraged us, directed us, and created opportunities for us to give shows even if it was just in our own living room in front of visitors. We loved doing it and it planted the seed of my lifelong love of musical theatre, which allowed me to combine my natural ability to create characters with singing and dancing. Things got more complicated when my father entered us in a talent show individually rather than as a sister act. Kathy sang "Honey Bun" from *South Pacific* while the more cerebral "A Wonderful Guy" was chosen for me. I won the individual song performance trophy and my sister won the overall show award so we both went home happy.

At age eleven, while our family was stationed in Turkey, I won the role of Helen Keller in the American high school production of *The Miracle Worker* and fell in love with theatre. Unlike many actors, it was not the approval and adoration of the audience that motivated me. I didn't want to "take them home with me." It was the character I was interested in, the work. Becoming someone other than myself for a short while was rewarding beyond anything else I had ever experienced. Thus I chose theatre as a major in college, not music. I still performed in and choreographed musicals, but it was the plays that fascinated me.

When I was in my thirties, it was film that captured my attention and, in particular, the documentary format. It wasn't just that so many more people could be exposed to the work, but also that it could be seen without having to perform it live over and over again. I had come to realize that theatre patrons were not my target audience. I was interested in what happened in living rooms on home entertainment systems where anyone could become the audience. Work that could be discussed, stopped, started, and viewed multiple times.

What attracted me to documentary work was my belief that real life is almost always more interesting and enlightening than fiction. I was fascinated by entering the world of different groups of people, allowing others to learn something they would otherwise never have the opportunity to experience. Mostly, I loved the idea of giving a collective voice to a group of people, people who for some reason could not find their own voice. I spent several years working on *Home of the Brave* about the plight of Vietnam veterans suffering trauma not just from their war experiences but from the terrible pain of coming home to a country that rejected them for what they were asked to do and did to the best of their ability. They suffered from Post Traumatic Stress Disorder (PTSD), similar to so many abuse victims. I felt a kinship with the veterans and was deeply committed to helping tell their story. I loved how hard they worked to find a way to be productive and overcome the enormous challenges they faced every day of their lives. I loved how they discovered at my urging that people really did care about them despite their fears of being rejected by the American people one more time. Mostly I loved how very grateful they were for having the opportunity to find their voices, something they assumed would never happen in their lifetime. I saw the transformation that was possible.

I watched young women in their 20's hear their own stories, as if for the first time, as they sat for interviews for my fourth documentary, *She Said.* It was empowering for them even to be asked how they felt and even more so to tell. A woman who worked for a major university health service told me that she believed the legacy of this generation of women was that they would "blow the lid off" their own stories, bring things out into the open and shine a bright light on their lives, even and especially the sad and tragic parts.

I wrote two screenplays and felt the enormous frustration of being unable to put together a financing deal to get the films made. It was difficult relying on so many other people to accomplish the simple goal of telling the story.

Recently, as my father's health began to fail, I realized that I was really telling my own story over and over again. The greatest work of my life had been overcoming the sexually abusive environment in which I was raised and the profound negative impact it had on my life. The emotional run-up to what my friend Andria calls "tumor day," my transformational bone marrow transplant, and the careful construction of a new, healthy life is a story I had been living and molding and creating my entire life. It was more powerful than any other story I could ever tell, it was something I knew from deep inside, and it was most likely shared by millions of other women, each with their own particular details but similar consequences. I had dedicated my life to discovering the meaning of my own story and began to believe that if I could find my own voice then maybe we, as a community of women, could find our collective voice. A voice of empowerment and strength filled with self-esteem and love. This truth would be my most profound work of art.

I could never have recreated what happened to me for this

book if I had not kept a detailed and ultimately lifesaving journal throughout the years that led to my cancer diagnosis. My emotional life was so overwhelming, so conflicted and so dangerous during that time that the only way I could keep from being swallowed whole by it was to write everything down. I wrote as a natural survival instinct. The words, once they hit the page, left my consciousness to make way for the next chapter. I had to make sure I cleared them out fast enough because if I ran out of space inside, the overcrowding would have smothered me to death. It was almost predictable that I would have to find a more permanent place for all those miserable feelings.

My enormous tumor, appropriately located in the female part of my body that interested my father when he molested me and later fascinated his surrogate, ultimately provided a place to house my sexual abuse and everything that came with it. It led to my transformational rebirth in a sterile bone marrow transplant room. And still I wrote. This time there were fewer words, raw words seeped in medical procedures, physical misery and hope.

There were lessons learned along the way that became the texture of my new, healthy life. I learned to say no, I learned to care for myself, I learned to allow myself to be loved, I learned to decide for myself who I wanted to be, I learned to choose what I wanted each and every day over and over, I learned to give up my need to control, and I learned to never let anyone control me ever again.

Abuse is very much like cancer. You have to go looking for it to see if it is causing trouble inside you. Both like to hide and stay undetected for as long as possible, burrowing their way inside you until you know something is terribly wrong, but through the art of denial, you don't even try to discover what it may really be. When your behaviors are out of control, when your body is screaming at you, when you can no longer manage your life, you will find cancer and/or abuse whether you want to or not. To me, they ultimately looked like one and the same. I knew for sure that they both had to be completely eliminated so I joined them together in the form of a breast tumor, and beat them mercilessly with chemotherapy, love, hope and faith. The way I look at it, if you have cancer or abuse or both, you'd better go looking for them because left unchecked, they will kill you. If not your body, certainly your soul.

I give you my story with tender care, the most precious gift I have to give. I spared nothing in the telling, believing in your ability to face it head on as I did. In my story, I hope you will find something that can be molded and shaped to have meaning for you. There is no other reason to share it than this hope. The power of the truth, no matter how painful, is our biggest weapon in healing. Use it, believe in it, resonate to it, champion it and learn to live within it. It will never let you down.

—Trish Kinney
Silver Platter Girl

SILVER PLATTER GIRL

PART ONE

EVERYTHING BEFORE

CHAPTER ONE

When I was born on St. Patrick's Day, three things weren't as planned. I had a large red birthmark that covered my entire right hand and arm, as well as part of my chest and back. Mammy, my paternal grandmother, said it was God's mark on me, the result of lightning that shocked my mother at seven months pregnant while turning on a light during a thunder storm in Mammy's living room in Sumter, South Carolina. Secondly, I was a girl. Not Thomas Daniel, the prior named boy I was destined to be. There already was a girl child, my sister Kathy. Without a girl's name planned for me, they chose the feminine version of St. Patrick, named me Patricia, and called me Patti. Finally, I had two different colored eyes, one brown and one blue.

During our many visits to Mammy's house throughout our childhood, we learned the Southern way. Dinner was at lunch, usually fried chicken with steamed rice and biscuits served on the pretty plates with the big pink flowers. Lunch was supper, in the early evening, lighter fare. We were allowed to lick the bowl when Mammy made a cake but only if we sat under the kitchen table. Our uncle worked at the Pepsi Cola bottling company so there were always wooden crates filled with Pepsi bottles around. You could grab one ice cold out of the fridge, pry off the top with a bottle opener, and the first swig would make your eyes sting.

On special occasions, my father would let me go with him to visit Mrs. Bernshouse. A large, kind woman in a full apron, she made desserts out of her big kitchen. The house always smelled delicious and if our chocolate roll, her specialty, wasn't quite ready when we arrived, I got to swing on the front porch while we waited to take it home warm from the oven.

Mammy never missed her favorite soap, "As the World Turns," in the afternoon and read us a Bible passage every evening before bed. She was famous for telling the story of the "crooked mouth family," mostly on short road trips, making us laugh so hard we cried no matter how many times we heard it. We picked up her perfect Southern drawl as soon as we arrived, gave it up just as quickly when we would leave, but got it right back every time we visited Sumter.

My father wanted to be a major league baseball player like his hometown hero, Bobby Richardson, a New York Yankee. Lacking in sufficient talent, his second choice was to fly, right out of Sumter. He enlisted in the Air Force and had to force feed bananas immediately prior to his physical so he could make the minimum weight. He went to Officer's Candidate School and became a fighter pilot. He met my mother in Bangor, Maine, where she was working at the Air Force base. They knew each other for a very short time before he proposed. Even though he got so drunk on their first date at the Officer's Club that he passed out head first onto his steak, she agreed. She was nineteen years old and broke her engagement with another man to run off with my father to see the world.

I took my first cross-country road trip at twelve weeks old with my sister and parents to the Grand Canyon. This was after a side trip to Duke University just long enough for the doctors there to tell my parents that some babies with birthmarks had been aggressively treated with radiation to lessen the wine colored stain but their arms stopped growing for good, leaving them with one infant-sized arm the rest of their life. The doctor's advice was to take me home, be glad I was healthy, and love me. My father enjoyed telling that story, as if explaining why he didn't find a way to make it go away and proving that he tried. Throughout my childhood, he assured me that God had personally given me this mark for a reason. He didn't tell me what that reason was and I didn't figure it out until much later. When I was five years old, I have a vivid memory of vowing to stay awake all night praying my hardest, absolutely certain that by morning God would have miraculously removed the stain from my body. I only nodded off a few times, but God decided against granting me my wish. This was the beginning of a kind of secular, spiritual faith that he offered me instead.

CHAPTER TWO

When we were assigned to a tour of duty in Holland, we traveled by ship. My mother was so seasick that she carried around a brown paper bag with an apple in it the entire time, the only food she could keep down. We lived in a Dutch house with a Dutch housekeeper. For my third birthday, I got a blue and white miniature china tea set. I insisted on carrying the tray upstairs to my room all by myself after the party was over, and dropped it on the first stair, shattering the cups and saucers. I was devastated and cried my eyes out. My sister's memories were more vivid.

Our house is small, neat and mostly wooden like the funny shoes people wear, like the big windmills high in the air, all through the countryside. Even our floors and the stairs inside are wooden.

Patti is only two. I am five years old. My sister is my best and only friend and we play together all the time, because even though I'm old enough for kindergarten, there isn't one.

At the top of the wooden stairs are two rooms. On the left is our playroom with no furniture, so we can play with our toys on the wooden floor, pretending together about all kinds of things. There are no books. Light shines in the windows, and it's the best room in our house. On the right is the bedroom where we sleep at night in twin beds.

Patti and I always take our bath together in the big tub with the claw feet, laughing and playing, singing and talking. Even though she is only two, my little sister is very smart. She listens to me a lot and likes it when I teach her things. I love to be her teacher and we play school.

Daddy teaches us nursery rhymes. He is leader of the songs at the grown-up parties and sings the loudest of everyone.

"Mary Ann Barnes was queen of all the acrobats
She could do tricks that would give a cat the fits"
"I love a billboard, I always will
Because a billboard gave me my first thrill
When I was just a little child, a sexy billboard drove me
wi—iii—ld"

We are very lucky because our Mommy is so beautiful and glamorous. Everybody says so. She wears pretty things, combs her hair a lot, and her lips are sticked all the time. She doesn't seem to mind at all when Patti and I watch her dressing up before her mirror in the morning and again just before night.

My favorite part is the way she puts on her bra, leaning over, wiggling into it, straightening up tall, tugging and lifting up the cups with both hands. My sister and I can see her fat teenie weenies, which are very important to her beautifulness. That's for sure. Her teenie weenies are the only fat part of her.

I can hardly wait to grow up as tall as my Mommy and especially to have fat teenie weenies like hers, so Daddy and all the boys will love mine like they love hers. Mine are just teenie weenies, not at all fat yet. I guess it will be quite a while before mine get fat like hers and Patti doesn't seem to care that much about them. She thinks Mommy's fat ones are funny. But, of course, she's only two.

Daddy goes on fighter pilot trips and brings back surprises for us. One time Mommy goes on a trip with him and we get the best present of all. We each get our very own bottle of pink fingernail polish! We have so much fun painting our fingers pink in the light of the playroom. Glamorous, like Mommy.

Sometimes my sister and I are allowed to go down to the living room parties late at night. We say hello to their friends. My favorite is called Davy Crockett, who is tall and handsome, just like the king of the wild frontier, and he treats me like I'm pretty special.

I also like Mommy's best friend whose name is Jackie, exactly the same as hers! But this Jackie is kind of fat all over, not just her teenie weenies, and looks like an opera star, and even sings just like an opera star with a rose in her teeth. She has a little boy named Frankie, who is my first friend, besides my sister.

Patti and I are allowed to sing our nursery rhymes for the grown ups. They clap for us and make us feel like movie stars. Then we go back upstairs, back to sleep in our twin beds.

Sometimes we take very long baths upstairs while the grown-ups are laughing and singing downstairs. Once a man comes in the bathroom while my sister and I are playing and washing in the tub, and he looks a little surprised to see us, but doesn't say anything. Instead, he just goes to the potty, standing up. My sister is really scared and almost cries, but I tell her to be very quiet and we stay frozen still, we don't splash or make any noise, and then he finishes and leaves the bathroom. We don't tell.

They have lots of grown-up parties, mostly at our house, when Daddy isn't on a fighter pilot trip. But sometimes Mommy gets really dressed up and they go out to other places. Cocktail parties, they're called. Our Dutch maid won't come to our house at night. So we are dressed in our jammies and jackets at party time and we go to the base nursery. My sister and I really hate to go there. We cry and cry and beg them not to take us there. But they do anyway.

It's a huge drafty room and very dark because all the lights are off except at the front check in counter where Mommy and Daddy leave us. There's no place to play, which doesn't matter because it's bedtime when we go there, no matter what time it is. The room is filled with long straight rows of small cots, very close together. Each cot is just alike, with white sheets and a pillow, and a scratchy green army blanket.

The grown-ups in charge are very mean about making all us kids be quiet, because it's time to go to sleep. They won't even read us stories and we're not allowed to talk.

Nearly every cot has a kid in it, but we don't know any of them. They are small American kids whose parents must be going to the same party. We whisper but the mean grown-ups tell us to be quiet and go to sleep right now. We both cry as softly as we can and then fall asleep with our faces in the pillows. It is very scary and I try to make sure my sister's cot is right next to mine. The base nursery is a terrible place. We hate it.

Much later that night, or when it's still dark and cold in the morning, they come for us. Mommy goes to Patti's cot, I guess because my sister is smaller and easier to carry sleeping to the car.

Daddy comes to my cot and stays a long time while Mommy and my sister wait in the car. He wakes me up, slowly and strangely, smelling like those party cocktails.

After the base nursery, I don't look at my eyes in the mirror anymore. I don't know why.

From Holland, we moved to Germany where we lived in a large apartment building reserved for American service families. There were small quarters in the building's basement for the German maids. Hanna Laura Klink was nice to us girls but I remember my Mom being mad at her a lot, accusing her of stealing her bras and underwear. She would send my Dad down to her room in the basement to talk to her about it and see if he could find the stolen goods. He seemed happy to do it and often stayed down there quite a while. My maternal grandmother, Grandlady, visited once and brought matching flannel nightgowns that she had made for me and my sister. Unfortunately, the wrist elastic was too tight and we woke up with hands swollen twice their normal size. One night while laying in my bed in the dark, I calmly and deliberately ate several plastic pop beads for no particular reason. The doctor said they would pass.

CHAPTER THREE

Upon our return to the States, we took up residence on a little radar site in Northern California called Point Arena. Base housing consisted of 27 small look alike units with carports. Once while spending the night with a little girl and her family, I got so homesick that I made my friend wake her mom at 2 am so I could ask her to call my parents to come get me. In a comfy robe with her very long hair pulled back in a ponytail tied low at the nape of her neck, she cradled me on her lap in the dark living room and showed me how her hearing aid worked. Despite her loving efforts to distract me, I begged her to make the call and I went home.

When I started school in the tiny town's only first grade class, I was ahead of the other students because my sister had taught me to read over the summer. My split class consisted of four rows of first graders and two rows of second graders. At mid-year, Mrs. Scarmella suggested that I move my first grade desk to join the second graders on the far side of the room closest to the window so the work would be more challenging for me. She explained that even though the front of my report card said Grade 1, she would fill in the back page saying, "This student is promoted to Grade 3" instead of Grade 2. Since we were moving after the school year anyway, she felt hardly anyone would even notice and if they did, it could be easily explained. My parents agreed. By the time

I was "unofficially" promoted to third grade, Mrs. Scarmella was expecting twins. We moved away before they were born.

So I slipped right into third grade when we moved to Beale Air Force Base in Marysville, California. At first we lived in a house whose best feature was its proximity to a grand indoor roller skating rink. Kathy and I spent all our free time there and had matching reversible skating skirts although we always chose to wear the black corduroy side up with the white satin underneath. I was beside myself when we found a pair of used white leather roller skates someone had outgrown that fit me perfectly so I no longer had to skate in the rentals.

One evening, Kathy and I were taking a bubble bath together and my Mom came in and found us posing provocatively, elbows up, hands behind our heads. She asked us what we were doing and I said we were playing Playboy playmates. Horrified by this admission that we had ever even seen a Playboy magazine, much less that we were emulating its models, she called my father in and sternly reprimanded him for keeping his Playboy magazines in the house where we could find them. He seemed to love our little game, grinning from ear to ear.

Once we moved to the base, my sister and I formed the Fillies Club with our best friend and neighbor, Robin, based on our love of horses. We adopted the names Diamond Storm, the Flame, and Satan, composed and often sang our Fillies anthem, raised money for the treasury by washing cars, and collected horse statues. That same summer we learned sign language. On my birthday, I got a sea green portable typewriter along with a typing instruction manual. Within a short time, I could type 35 words per minute mostly using the practice sentence "They urged her to get the right dried fruit there."

I got called to the office one day at school to meet with a man who asked me a lot of questions. The school then asked my parents' permission to give me an IQ test to determine whether I should skip another grade. This time it was clear to me that even though my father allowed my mother to weigh in on this decision, it was his to make. And he seemed to like the idea. On the day of the test, I knew I was performing miserably. I expressed my anxiety to my father later that evening and asked him the answers to all the questions I wasn't sure about. He went over each of them with me, which somehow made me feel better. But I was right about the results and the school was quite surprised at my poor showing on the test. I was determined to have a second chance and prove that people were not wrong about me. Remembering that during the test someone asked us to pick up and move to another room, I proclaimed that it was upsetting to be interrupted in the middle of the test and the disruption had negatively affected my performance. A retest was scheduled. To my amazement, they gave me the exact same test so my father's answers assured my success. It was decided that it would be best for me to move across the courtyard mid-year to the fifth grade classroom and get as much out of fourth and fifth grade in one school year as I could. The problem was I missed the second half of fourth grade curriculum and the first half of fifth. I was terrified when I had to leave my old room to join a classroom full of older strangers who had lunch and recess at a different time. By now I was two years younger than my classmates and only one grade behind my sister who was three years my senior. I heard my parents whispering that there would be no more grade skipping.

CHAPTER FOUR

In sixth grade, I fell in love with Tommy Ognisty at McClellan Air Force Base near Sacramento. He lived across the street so we got to see each other all the time. We were inseparable. I felt very nervous about my physical attraction to him, not sure if that was allowed or something you could get in trouble for. Once we went to a baseball game together and he pulled me close to him, leaning me against his legs and putting his hands on my shoulders. I asked my Mom what she thought about it. For the life of me, I cannot remember her answer but I know she didn't discourage it or think it was naughty.

By this time my sister and I were taking piano lessons and had a singing act. We performed a medley from the *Sound of Music* that we arranged ourselves at a school recital. My mother was rehearsing a dancing role for an Officers' Wives Club musical production of *The Drunkard*. As a child she had been known as Baby Jackie Anderson, tap dancing up and down a set of little wooden stairs, an act once featured on the *Major Bowes Amateur Hour*, the popular radio show. There was a small speaking role for a young girl about my age in the show, daughter of the drunkard. They were having trouble casting the role and had reluctantly given it to the girl who lived across the street, a friend of mine. The only problem was she was very chubby and did not fit the part of a poor waif whose no good father had deserted the family, leaving them penniless. My mother informed the director that her daughter was very tiny, a good actress with performing experience, beyond her years in maturity and education, and prepared to take on the role. After my audition, Jill was told that she no longer had the part and it was given to me. My excitement over winning the role was overshadowed by sadness for my friend and I was amazed that she still agreed to play with me.

My father was called away in the summer of 1962 for several weeks and we were not allowed to know where he was, later learning he had been involved with the Cuban missile crisis. We were told that his next assignment would be for one year in Thule, Greenland, a solo tour. Horrified at the thought of ice cold Greenland, he negotiated a different deal. We would all go to Ankara, Turkey for two and a half years. This meant I had to say goodbye to Tommy Ognisty, which broke my heart. We listened to our song, "See You in September," over and over knowing full well we would never see each other again.

CHAPTER FIVE

After a stop in Sumter to visit Mammy, and six weeks in Washington DC for Turkish language and culture school, we left for Turkey. Every incoming family had an advisor family that helped in finding a place to live, getting settled and learning the ropes. Our new home was the entire third floor of a four story apartment building on a small street off Cunkaya Hill. It had three bedrooms, a big living room and dining room and a balcony on two sides. Kathy and I shared the sunny bedroom with a side balcony and plenty of room for the two of us. The Turkish handyman who lived in the basement lugged our big drinking water jugs all the way up the stairs on his shoulder, all vegetables had to be soaked in Clorox before eating, and we could brush our teeth with tap water if we promised not to swallow. The landlord's family lived on the top floor and spoke no English. Their daughter, Hatije, a pretty girl in her late teens with black hair and dark mischievous eyes, had a crush on my Dad. We could see the Russian Embassy from our balcony, an ominous, heavily secured property that scared the living daylights out of us. One day in late November, Hatije's mother came rushing hysterically down the stairs to our apartment yelling Kennedy, boom boom, with a single finger pointing at her temple. We had no television or radio so it took us a while to confirm that President Kennedy had been shot. We watched from our balcony as the Russians gathered excitedly on the roof of their embassy.

One evening my father brought home the *Stars and Stripes* newspaper and said he wanted to show us something funny. There on the top of an inside page was a photograph of the Beatles with their long hair. My father proclaimed them to be a gimmick that wouldn't last. Every time the Base Exchange got a shipment of new records, we clamored to get there early enough to buy the latest Beatle album, which came straight from England on the Parlophone label. We listened to the songs over and over again on our small battery operated record players. When the BX could not keep up with our voracious appetite for all things Beatles, Grandlady would buy the newest 45s in the States and ship them to us. Even Christmas morning could not compare with the delirium of ripping open the package to find a copy of "I Saw Her Standing There" inside.

My sister and I expanded our singing act to include the Riddle sisters, Pat and Judy. They were exactly our ages and our parents became very close friends as well. They lived a little further up the hill in easy walking distance, which was important because we didn't have telephones. I could take the shortcut up the narrow dirt path behind our house but I had to run my fastest, scared to death, past the little shack where the one-eyed man with the disfigured face and hunched back lived. We had all heard the rumors of the band of gypsies that kidnapped children in the city and took them to the hills to live the vagabond life, never to be heard from again. I was sure the beggar in the shack was the lookout for the gypsies and was planning to snatch me any day. Judy and I would stay overnight together, mostly at her house because she had a double bed. We had a back scratcher and would give each other long turns on our backs, arms and legs well into the night. We once had a conversation as to which part of our bodies we would expose if forced to expose only one, our breasts or down there. She immediately said she would expose her breasts but I was adamant that I would choose the lower part rather than let someone see my breasts even though there was yet no evidence of breasts on my tiny, immature body. Our families vacationed together at isolated Turkish beaches, often barely accessible by car, where camels roamed the shore and more than once we sang in local restaurants and bars. We visited Athens, Greece where Judy, Pat, Kathy and I were allowed to have our own hotel room.

Our school was a big, very old purple warehouse in the city, a temporary facility until the new school was completed. I was inducted into the National Honor Society as a junior high student there, allegedly the youngest ever to be chosen as a result of my grade skipping. Each of the inductees wore a white shirt with dark pants or skirts, and held a candle that was lit by an existing NHS member. The new school had a dorm to accommodate American kids from all over Europe because their families were stationed in places that didn't have schools.

One day the French teacher, a black man, stopped me in the hall and asked me to come with him to an empty classroom. Without even turning on the lights, he asked me to throw a desk across the room as hard as I could to determine my strength and fortitude. Then, as director, he offered me the role of Helen Keller in the school production of *The Miracle Worker*. What followed was a grueling four-month rehearsal period for which the chair throwing did not prepare me. Most of the time I was blindfolded, which helped me relate to Helen's extreme disability but once caused me to fall off the second story bedroom open set piece and often sent me home with bumps and bruises from banging into furniture. There were times I wanted to quit out of sheer exhaustion and emotional fatigue. It didn't help that Judy only had a small role so we weren't able to spend time together as we usually did since I was always rehearsing or doing homework. My teachers complained to my parents that rehearsals were interfering with my schoolwork and they hoped things would improve when it was all over. The show was a hit in its short run at our new school and I remember a lady sending my parents a hand written note saying I was a "budding Sarah Bernhardt." Soon after, life returned to normal.

Judy and I rode horses and were allowed to take the bus to the stables in the lower part of the city by ourselves. She was the better, more daring rider and felt comfortable on the temperamental horses. I preferred Atil, the biggest, gentlest horse in the stable. We took lessons and learned to jump over small fences. A Turkish shoemaker measured my feet and made custom black leather riding boots for me. We had to order my jodhpurs from a riding catalogue and it was very hard finding them small enough to fit me. They still had to be taken in when they arrived. My father went to Paris on business and brought me a beautiful riding hat, black velvet with white satin lining. He also brought white French jeans and brightly colored stretchy tank tops to all three of his girls.

Around this time, my parents decided that Kathy, being a teenager now, would no longer share a room with me and they would fix up the smaller, drearier middle bedroom for her. My mother tried to make it nice and had a white wrought iron glass top dressing table made for her but the room never really came together. The funny thing was that my sister never asked for her own room; she just got it anyway. We were sad at being separated that way. I missed her.

One evening, my father agreed to take us down to the American movie theatre. Believing we were going to see a family film, he dropped us off and left. Instead it was an adult film, *In the French Style*, and we had no way to contact my Dad to come back and get us. I refused to go in at first, telling Kathy we would definitely not be allowed to see such a movie. She insisted and told me to stop being such a baby. As the movie's adult sexual theme developed, I hid my eyes and demanded that we leave and wait for Dad upstairs in the base library. Kathy wouldn't hear of it even though I was completely traumatized by the sexual openness of the film, knowing absolutely nothing about the subject but knowing this was not how I wanted to learn about it. What surprised me was that my sister seemed to know a lot about the subject. When we got home, I was terribly upset and clung to my mother knowing that she would understand my indignation at having been subjected to this completely inappropriate experience. She decided that it was immediately necessary for my father to sit us both down in the living room and give us "the talk" about the birds and the bees. She was making dinner but it was all put on hold for this big family event. My father seemed overly excited about this task assigned to him by my mother and couldn't stop grinning, an expression I had seen only once before on the day we were caught playing Playboy playmates in the tub. She interrupted him several times when she deemed his choice of words inappropriate or out of line. My sister squirmed and seemed dark and distraught. I thought she was just really mad at me for telling about seeing the wrong movie and getting us into all this. Whatever the cause, I had a very bad feeling.

My parents went on a trip to Brussels to celebrate their anniversary. One day after school, I came across a box of slides of the photos they had taken on their trip. Anxious to see what Brussels was like, I began looking at the slides, shocked to find the photos were of my mother in her bikini bottom without her top on, smiling seductively. I was very upset seeing her that way. She said it was ok for a husband and wife to do things like that in private. I said it wasn't private if I saw it. She said I shouldn't have opened the box of pictures without permission. I said who could have guessed it wouldn't be ok.

Gradually I became known as the high-strung child with the nervous stomach. I was just beginning to discover that I had the ability to take on the symptoms and experiences of others as if they were my own. There was a new boy in school who had polio and couldn't walk without crutches, dragging his lifeless legs behind. I would lie in my bed at night and declare that my legs were paralyzed. I created many other physical symptoms, often manifesting themselves as stomach problems. No doctor could find a thing wrong with me. But I felt sick a lot.

My father continued to mentor me as the proud parent of a smart kid. He suggested important books for me to read that no one else would ever offer to a child my age. And I read them. When I expressed a fear of flying to my oral surgeon appointments in Germany or the dentist in Athens, he got out his flight manual and explained to me in scientific terms what made a plane stay suspended in the air and why it was safer than getting in a car. He showed me how to read the stock market page of the paper and together we tracked his small investments. My mother put her foot down when he wanted to teach me how to balance the family checkbook, saying their finances were none of my business. She almost seemed mad at me. He relished my good grades and took great pride in the attention heaped on me for my performing abilities. He told me never to settle for being a nurse when I could be the doctor, or a stewardess when I could fly the plane. He never put it in the context of my being a girl; instead it was always that I was plenty smart to be whatever I wanted. I gradually came to understand that this was my place in the family, in his world. He didn't talk to my sister in the same way. She seemed to have a different place, although I had no idea what it was. I don't remember my dad hugging me or tucking me in at night or ever even pulling me onto his lap for a cuddle. He held me in a different way. I learned to treasure my brain as my best asset and my best protector.

My sister and I grew apart after she got her own room. I heard rumors that she went on a school camping trip and did whatever the boys wanted. She was angry at me a lot, calling me Patti Perfect and accusing me of telling on her all the time. It was hard to understand because we had been best friends all our lives as we moved from place to place and had only one another to play with and confide in. We had spent hours in highly competitive games of double solitaire and contests to see who could walk on their hands the longest. But those days were gone. She once called me a "pukey ferd" while heading downstairs to catch the bus on a rainy day. I stopped in my tracks and ran back upstairs to tell my mom, who put her on restriction. I see now where that would have infuriated my sister. But she was no longer the sister I knew.

Now that our time in Turkey was almost up, we had orders for Colorado Springs where Robin, the former Filly, and her family were living and we could have real horses. But as the movers were loading our boxes on the truck, we got a TWIX from some military authority saying our orders had been changed to the Pentagon. My father was most unhappy about it but this time, he could not talk his way out of it. We didn't know at the time that my sister was taking a case of Turkish tuberculosis home to the States with us.

CHAPTER SIX

It was like a dream arriving in the US where we had phones, televisions, transistor radios, shopping malls and American neighbors. We bought a brand new split-level Colonial in Canterbury Woods that I heard my parents say we couldn't afford but was in the best school district. We paid $28,900 for it. We had to live in a small two-bedroom apartment while the house was being built. Kathy and I shared a room again. Every night we fell asleep to the Beatles' *Rubber Soul* album played on the battery operated record player on the table between our beds. It was a good feeling being together again, familiar, even though it was only for a few months. She seemed more like her old self somehow, and we enjoyed sharing a bedroom.

I entered W. T. Woodson High School as a freshman at twelve years old, well under five feet tall, and sixty-nine pounds. I was told on more than one occasion that the junior high was just behind the building and I must have wandered into the wrong school. When I was in the office registering, they asked me if I liked to be called Patricia or something else. With no warning, I was stunned to hear the word "Trish" come out of my mouth. "They call me Trish," I said. When I left the office and walked down the hall, one of the secretaries called out to me, and I didn't even turn around when she repeated my new name several times. I must not have mentioned this renaming of myself to my parents. When I received my first phone call at home, the caller asked for Trish and my mother said they must have the wrong number. She didn't take the news well and insisted, to no avail, that I go back to my real name, Patti. My father supported my show of independence and accommodated by calling me by my new name right away.

In the new house, I had a small room of my own with wood floors and a tiny closet. For Christmas one year, I got the white canopy bed of my dreams along with a purple area rug and matching lavender floral bedspread and canopy. That year, Kathy's best friend, Marsha, whom we called Shashee, one of the prettiest, most popular girls in our high school, gave me the Beatles' *White Album*. I listened to it for hours at a time, looking out the one small window in my room from my bed at the moon or sometimes the snow falling in the halo of the streetlight on the corner.

My sister began to experience a pain in her chest that wouldn't go away. After various tests, she was diagnosed with tuberculosis. There was talk of sending her away for treatment and recovery, but my mother would have none of it. Instead she agreed to a grueling regimen of keeping my sister's clothes and dishes separate from ours, disinfecting her things, and keeping up with her various medications including daily shakes to try to keep weight on her. She wore a mask whenever she left her room. The school district provided a speaker system, one in Kathy's room and one carried from class to class at school by friends. She was able to complete her studies, staying on track to graduate with her class the following year. I developed the same exact chest pain, absolutely certain I, too, had the disease.

When Kathy began to recover and was cleared to rejoin the world, her relationship with my mother began to change. They argued a lot and disagreed on most everything. My mother was always accusing my sister of something and disapproved of the way she dressed. One day my sister put on shorts and a yellow tank top with a push up bra, although being willowy thin, she didn't have a lot to show off. My mother became enraged and yelled that she was not going out dressed in that top. She instructed my father to "take care of it." Standing in the doorway of my room watching this unfold, I noticed that he seemed extremely uncomfortable intervening between his wife and his daughter on this particular subject. But he put his foot down as asked, telling my sister to go to her room and change her outfit immediately. Kathy looked betrayed, which I remember seemed like an odd thing in and of itself, and stood her ground, refusing to obey. He walked towards her, backing her into the hall bathroom, and slapped her hard across the face, sending her running past him to her room in tears.

Unlike my sister, I still had a very immature body and it was especially difficult to compete in high school with girls who already looked like women. It cost me a spot on the cheerleading squad, which I deserved. I had to buy my clothes in the children's department, a perfect girls 6X. Out of necessity, I learned to sew and began creating my own fashion style featuring very short dresses, colored stockings and Capezio leather shoes. The girls' PE teacher, a tough woman, routinely threatened to send me to the office because my skirts were too short and finally suggested that I just add a ruffle to the hem of every one of them.

Many years of dance training had paid off and I was doing well in the Modern Dance Club. One day a talented student had been instructed by his art teacher to wander the halls looking for things to sketch. He swears that it was love at first sight when he looked in the modern dance rehearsal room and saw me dancing on a table, and Michael became the first boy since Tommy Ognisty who made me feel safe and loved. He was very careful with me, very patient, and waited in the background when I wanted to experiment with racier boys who were starting to occasionally pay attention to me. But he was always there. One day he rang my doorbell with a small box in his hand. It was a dainty promise ring with two small diamond chips. I accepted it, wore it on my right hand, and he expected nothing in return.

My closest friend, Marianne, was making plans to move to California just as the Mamas and Papas' song, "California Dreaming," was hitting the charts. She had a boyfriend, Pete, a hunky swimmer who adored her. When she left, we were both inconsolable and Pete, in his depressed, miserable state, turned his affections to me. Of course I was just a substitute for her but he was such a status symbol that I willingly went along. He invited me to his senior prom and I was devastated beyond belief when my parents said they would not allow me to go with him due to our age difference. He was already a year ahead of me in school, which made him three years older than me and after all, I was only fourteen. He couldn't be trusted, they said, and I was just too young to be put in that position. I argued relentlessly that it was just a school dance, but they knew what unseemly things were likely to take place after the dance was over and even though I promised I wouldn't take part in those things, they refused to change their minds. They even brought in a Catholic priest who was a family friend and agreed to defer to his judgment but he sided with them. I pointed out that it was they who had allowed me to skip two grades and it wasn't fair to expect me to bear up to the responsibility of that for all those years without allowing me the privileges that go along with it. What I thought was air tight bargaining was unsuccessful. It was the biggest disappointment of my young life. Pete was accepted at the Naval Academy and went off to Annapolis after graduation. He wrote love letters from the Academy and agreed to accompany me to my senior prom in his dress uniform. I made my pastel, empire waist dress from a Vogue pattern and wore long above the elbow white gloves. Michael was crushed.

My father had taken to coming into my room at night to "lay with me." He was not welcome at all, especially when he would throw his arm over my stomach and either fall asleep or pass out, I'm not sure which, as there was always drinking involved. I went to my mother to ask her to tell him that I didn't want him to do that anymore. She wouldn't. Well, she didn't.

I wasn't old enough to get my driver's license until right before graduation, about the time I started my period for the first time. All my friends were making college plans. My parents decided that I was too young to leave home. Our Pentagon tour was over and I was grateful that for the first time in my father's career, we had been allowed to stay put for four years, my entire high school career. He would be attending the Air Force War College in Montgomery, Alabama for one year before heading to Vietnam.

That summer, my family took a two-week beachfront rental in Myrtle Beach, South Carolina. Michael came to visit for a few days and we spent a carefree, innocent time holding hands, swimming in the ocean, and going to the amusement park in the evenings. When it was time for him to leave, I walked him to his car. Knowing how much he loved me, I was certain that he would speak to the future he envisioned, or at least desperately wanted, for us. I was nervous about it because no matter how comfortable and safe I felt with him, I knew there were many things I would have to face in my life, many things I would want to accomplish, that could not be done with him by my side. He was too sweet, too loving and would not have the stomach for the course my life would inevitably take even though I had no idea what that course would be. It was always hard for him to ask for what he wanted and his strong intuition as to what was best for me was almost always accurate despite how often it did not include what he wanted for himself. He planned every move very carefully. He intuitively knew that if he made any demands on me, asked for any commitments that day at the beach, I would have turned him down. And he was right. Still he surprised me by asking for nothing. I watched him drive away, knowing he was leaving me to my own future, one that would take place without him, even though that was not what he wanted. Little did I know that he would patiently wait for so many years to reenter my life and play such a significant part at such a critical time.

CHAPTER SEVEN

I enrolled in Huntingdon College, a private liberal arts school with a very small theatre department just a few miles from our rental home in a nice Montgomery neighborhood. Even though my father felt strongly that my choice of a major should be practical, my high school theatre teacher had convinced me that I should major in theatre. My parents bought me a little white Triumph Spitfire convertible and I commuted to campus in my trademark short skirts that barely passed the strict classroom dress code. As a member of the college dance group, the Huntingdon Honeys, I performed on a regular basis. I was even offered a job teaching the college ballet classes for school credit, in charge of and giving grades to students years older than myself. My role as Ado Annie in the spring musical, *Oklahoma*, made me a local celebrity, once receiving a standing ovation in a restaurant after a performance. I loved running with my theatre friends who were flamboyant and idealistic, often dancing at local clubs and splashing around in public fountains late at night. The only one I dated was gay, although he was not open about it at the time, so he prevented our relationship from getting physical, which was puzzling for me. The baritone who had the lead in *Oklahoma* had a crush on me and once wrote about his tender feelings on the back of my Barbra Streisand poster. I would go into the very old, tiny theatre on campus from time to time and sing "I'm the Greatest Star" on stage all by myself, believing every word.

I tried to concentrate on my non-arts classes but it was extremely difficult. In particular I had a Tuesday-Thursday history class that I could barely make myself attend. I wrote:

History 102. . .2,4 (1:15)

Four cold walls, a roof, a floor
And hundreds of years of history
Bound and printed exquisitely
The Sun King rises, rules and sets
Charles had a head and then does not
While five circles of time escape
Rousseau comes forth, expounds, now rots
But his words caused the Bastille to fall
(Please star that)

Soldiers march along dusty roads
Dropping one by one
To the tune of a couple ticks and several tocks
And the world rejoices when its last war ends
Until the second one begins

Left is one blank page for us to fill
Space enough for 3 men and 4 dates
A stingy portion from a book so large
But when this page is filled, how will it be seen
By the future History Class 102. . .2,4 (1:15)

When my father graduated from the War College, Huntingdon offered me a full scholarship to stay the remaining three years but my parents still weren't ready to let me go. My mother and I got out a map of the United States to choose where we were going to live while my father was in Vietnam. We picked Phoenix, a place where my parents hoped to retire one day. I looked in the college catalogue and found out that Arizona State University had a good theatre department. We would take up residence there while he was gone.

There was a short summer stay in Sacramento, California, prior to his departure. I became friends with two boys in our cul-de-sac and spent every day with them. Right before I left, my parents let me drive up to San Francisco with them for the day. We had so much fun listening to the car radio and eating sourdough bread on the wharf. The morning I left, I found a note from one of them saying how much he cared for me. It was the perfect summer fling without a single kiss.

It was also the summer of Woodstock. I was completely captivated by the film as my political conscience began to stir. Using my own money, I bought the double album soundtrack and was very excited for my parents to hear Jimi Hendrix play the "Star Spangled Banner" on his guitar. They didn't take it well at all, my mother scratching the needle all the way across the record to make it stop. She lectured me on my father going to Vietnam to risk his life for our country asking how I could listen to something so disrespectful, making it perfectly clear it wouldn't be played in our home. Being a good patriot all my life, respecting my father's service, jumping out of the base pool at 5 pm on summer days to stand with hand over heart for the lowering of the flag, hearing the National Anthem before every movie at the base theatre, I did not consider Jimi's version disrespectful. How unfair I thought it was for her to make such an assumption. She banned the recording and I returned it to the store.

CHAPTER EIGHT

My father left for Southeast Asia and we drove to Phoenix. It was very, very hot and I was terrified of the rattlesnakes that in my vivid imagination were around every corner. We rented a townhouse in Tempe, near ASU, and made many friends right away. Most of our social life centered around the community pool, located right outside our front door. The day I went to register at the university, it must have been one hundred and ten degrees. Deeply tanned from hours spent at the pool, I couldn't help but notice that most of the other girls wore shorts and jeans while I was still wearing my Huntingdon dresses. It was so hot that I stopped on the walkway in front of gorgeous Gammage Auditorium, took off my sandals, and stood barefoot in the sprinklers to cool off my legs and feet. I had seen a picture of Gammage in the college catalogue and dreamed of performing there, a huge step beyond the small stage in the campus chapel at Huntingdon. I chose a monologue from *The Miracle Worker* for my audition, playing Annie Sullivan this time, and was accepted into the theatre department.

I had begun to attract attention from the opposite sex now that I was seventeen. I met a quiet, sensitive and handsome young man who also lived at the townhouses. His mother had moved the family to Tempe following the untimely death of her husband. We became very close and spent our evenings together, which gradually led to a physical relationship. He took it very slowly as we would walk to the park at night and kiss, sitting on the grass. He had nothing to do with my college life or my performing life, and we never went on dates. One night, he gently put his hand on my breast, the first time this had ever happened to me. I went into my mom's room after he left, woke her up, and told her. When his adorable, seventeen year old brother, Danny, was diagnosed with cancer and died, the family moved back to Montana. My life, as I knew it, was about to change dramatically, a result of my sister's upcoming marriage and the sexual attention of two men, both extremely dangerous and hard to resist for very different reasons.

CHAPTER NINE

Our townhouse community hired a University student as a part-time pool attendant. He wasn't a lifeguard, just someone to make sure the rules were followed and the kids stayed in line. The job seemed a perfect fit for him. He was Hispanic, a former local high school football hero, generally averse to hard work, but appropriately intimidating with his muscular physique to manage whatever situation came up. But his real interest seemed to be the women lying out at the pool in their bikinis. Me included. He had a sensual, secretive way about him that made you feel as though you were the sole object of his desire and he could not live without having you completely. He was open about it. It started very soon after we became acquainted. He invited me to a hotel room to have his way with me, on a daily basis, and never gave up trying. I was flattered and flustered by this sexual attention, which was completely new to me as I had never been propositioned before. At seventeen, I certainly wasn't considering his proposition, but imagined I could keep him on the hook at some level without actually having to "go all the way" which I had never done and had no intention of doing with him. There was one girl, a real blonde bombshell we called Purple Ramona. Her bikini, the color of which inspired her nickname, was small but she completely filled it out, spilled out of it. Our pool attendant had a special thing going with her. I really didn't want to know if they were having at it because that would somehow force me to face how unprepared I was to even play in this arena, how high the stakes were. She had a sense of entitlement, as though she had some level of control over him that we others didn't have. He looked at her in a particularly carnal way but it didn't stop him from constantly seeking out other options. Relentlessly.

One day our neighbor, Jean, who lived next door and served as the community Board President, told me how much they were enjoying having him around and what a good hire he turned out to be. She casually mentioned his wife and young daughter, which caused me to immediately summon my best acting skills to appear as if I already knew. I was stunned to discover he wasn't available after the manner in which he had been treating me. I was ashamed and angry. He wasn't too pleased when I confronted him, obviously hoping I would never find out, but didn't deny his situation. The pregnancy and marriage were the result of a high school romance and their strict Catholic upbringing dictated that they would marry and raise the child. I was amazed at how easy it was to forget about his family, even after Jean had shown me a photograph of his little girl, while he flirted, cajoled, and literally begged me to have sex with him. It was the first time I recognized my father in me and it was oh so easy to justify. James would make sure I knew his weekly work schedule and I would make sure I was available to sit by the pool or go into the clubhouse to shoot pool or just talk quietly for hours into the evening. He also found my mother attractive and enjoyed the idea that she and I lived alone waiting for my father to return from the war. It was he, for the first time, who made me feel my own sexual power. My father had taught me that a woman's control emanated from her sexuality, but it was never anything I could believe or relate to. Until James. Now I understood what my father meant, but still had no intention of accommodating James' increasingly desperate desire to seduce me. Day after day, he turned every comment into a sexual image, an invitation, a summons. What I don't think he counted on was that we would get to know each other, become close friends. His other "relationships" were hunt, conquer, and leave. Although I was certainly hunted, I wasn't to be conquered, and he wasn't leaving. How could I have known at the time that his persistent pursuit of me would lead directly to the most dangerous threat I would ever face, but would also create such a lifesaving and profound opportunity for transformative healing?

My sister, Kathy, was getting married. Her future husband had come to the door selling curb address painting services when we lived in Montgomery. He was a hometown boy with a sweet Southern drawl and she took to him right away. The wedding was to take place in Tempe and my father was taking a short leave from his tour in Southeast Asia to attend. I was the maid of honor. My mother was ecstatic with the excitement and anticipation of seeing my father after a separation of six months. She let me know how difficult it was for them to be apart without sex for that long and how important their sexual reunion would be. It wasn't unusual for her to speak openly about such things. She was also excited about my sister's wedding and enthusiastically made plans for the small event.

The November weekend arrived, as did everyone involved. My father seemed on top of the world to be home and fully engaged in the wedding events. I was a serious Barbra Streisand fanatic by this time and knew every song she had ever recorded. I often sang along with her records to anyone who would listen. The family favorite during this visit was "Happy Days are Here Again." My father brought me the Barbra Streisand Christmas Album, recorded live in Central Park, as a gift. I quickly headed to our older model Cadillac in the carport to listen because it was the only eight-track player we had. It was well into the evening, dark, and I was in ecstasy getting my first listen to the new album away from all the commotion going on inside. Listening to Barbra songs was a very private, almost religious experience to me. My father followed me to the car and slid into the passenger side. He had been drinking, as always by this time of night. I instantly had the same feeling as when he would come into my room in Virginia and "lay with me." It was like a freezing in my body, a fear of moving. It seemed best just to stay still until it passed. Only this time, it was different. With the Christmas music swelling, my father began to make out with me, just as any clumsy young boy would do at the drive-in on a date. He leaned in to kiss me sloppily and his hands began to roam across my chest, lingering on my right breast, but continually moving, almost in a rhythm. This molestation seemed oddly familiar to me even though he had never touched me in this way before. He seemed so comfortable with his technique, his approach, as though it came naturally to him. Confused and shocked, I reached for the door handle and fumbled my way outside of the car. I cannot remember where I went or how I got there. And I didn't tell anyone. I put it away, buried it, and went on as though it never happened.

My sister married the next day, my mother invited James to the reception, and I couldn't stop crying. When she left on her honeymoon, she seemed completely dazed and uncertain as to what was happening to her, almost like she was watching herself instead of participating. For the first time, I knew how that felt. I attended rehearsal for a show that evening, only barely able to manage the avalanche of emotion that continued to overwhelm me with no conscious understanding of its cause. I later learned that over that one weekend, my father had his sexual reunion with my mother, sat in the bathroom with my sister as she took her pre-wedding bath, introduced me to his sexual favors in the car, all the while looking forward to returning to his live-in lover at his flight base in Thailand.

CHAPTER TEN

When the school year was over, my father completed his tour in Vietnam and made plans to retire in Phoenix. He was offered a promotion to full Colonel if he would serve one final tour at Hanscom Field, outside of Boston. Reluctantly he agreed but only for the additional retirement benefits because he was anxious to be free of the bureaucracy of the military and start his new life. I was shocked to discover that my parents expected me to change schools once again and go with them, sticking to the increasingly tired excuse that I was still too young to be away from home. But I was now eighteen years old with a growing instinctive need for distance from my parents' marriage. They suggested Boston College, which was an appealing idea except that I would be commuting from the base every day, including returning home late at night after rehearsals. There would be no opportunity to live on campus and experience college life even though I would be a junior. It seemed exhausting and unsafe but they were blinded by their need to have me with them. I had never defied, disobeyed, or even barely disagreed with my parents. But I was dead set against attending three colleges in three years and was experiencing success as a theatre major at ASU. I announced that I would be returning to school in Arizona and would live in a small apartment near campus with a roommate, also a dancer. It was very difficult for me to find the nerve and the courage to be so assertive in my position as I wasn't nearly as confident as I pretended to be. I was scared and uncertain. On the day I left, my mother wept uncontrollably, still desperately trying to convince me it was a terrible mistake to leave home. I longed for their support and encouragement. It was a devastating experience.

My apartment, the Oasis, was across the street from campus and next door to a pancake house called Hobo Jo's, and the Dash Inn, a funky Mexican joint where I would later work. I rode my bike to class most days and had to lug it up and down three flights of stairs to my apartment. I dated an older guy, a construction contractor, who had a house close by. I would sometimes spend the night there on weekends at his request but never took off my bra and panties and never had sex with him. He bought a brand new silver Corvette and allowed me to drive it to rehearsal once. We sometimes went places in his pick up truck and I remember asking if I could look at his thick construction site notebook that was always on the front seat to learn more about his work. He shrugged off my request saying I would never understand it, in stark contrast with my father encouraging me to read his flight manuals to learn how planes stayed in the air. We drifted apart after that. I decided that I would never marry because no man could ever understand me and it was best if I just accepted that.

I began spending time with Tim, an artistic, gentle, fellow theatre student with a beautiful singing voice. He lived across the street in the old landmark teepee apartments. We did shows together and became very close. We decided we should probably make love, a first for both of us, and we discussed it incessantly. Should we or shouldn't we, we wondered with a nervous laugh. With neither of us knowing yet that he was gay, we often slept together in the same bed but never had sex. He won a role with the national touring company of *No, No, Nanette*, contracted AIDS and passed away very young.

James stayed in touch and never let up in his pursuit of me, arranging meetings on campus and often stopping by my apartment to visit. No longer seeing him daily at the townhouse pool helped keep my mind off him but I always chose my outfits carefully when I knew I would be seeing him for the sole purpose of driving him crazy. My efforts were obviously successful. He was crazy for me.

CHAPTER ELEVEN

The first time I laid eyes on my future husband was also the first time I intuitively knew anything for absolute sure. He lived five doors down from me and I went to the apartment mailboxes to find out his name. It was Dutch, two words. He was very tall, very long limbed, a natural blond with huge shoulders. With a golden tan and a quiet, thoughtful demeanor, he was simply the most gorgeous man I had ever seen. We visited in the pool where I learned he was from Iowa and attending law school at ASU. He wore gym trunks for swimming with nothing underneath which seemed perfectly natural. He didn't seem to notice my birthmark at all. And he didn't show a hint of lechery. The first time we went out together was a double feature at the drive in and he didn't even try to kiss me. We watched the movies. Once we took a drive out of town in his big red Buick with the white interior. I slid over on the bench seat to sit closer and he asked me to move back, saying he wasn't comfortable that way. He was naturally quiet, brilliant, and interested in everything I had to say, which was a lot. I nestled in to what was the safest place I had ever known.

To ensure my future, I had to knock on his door late at night when I would see the light on and invite him for a bike ride or ask to borrow an egg for a cake I wasn't really baking. I was going to spend the rest of my life with him. Rather quickly we were sexually active. Unlike the other men with whom I had contemplated sex, there was no need to think about it and decide whether I should or not. It was a given. It took me a while to learn the ropes of lovemaking and he didn't care a bit if my inexperienced and small body needed a lot of time and patience to get the hang of it. That summer he saw me perform in a big musical production at the University, a singing and dancing role in the musical *Company*. The first time he told me he loved me, he was almost amused that I seemed to make such a big deal of the moment. It was my first glimpse into the steady security and natural acceptance of being loved by a Dutch man. We didn't have to talk about it so much. It just was, once it was. And that was all there was to it.

My parents came into town and we had dinner with them. If there was any doubt in my mind at the time that Mark was my life partner, it was erased after that dinner. He completely understood my father. He recognized how controlling, how bright, how manipulative, how easily titillated, and how inappropriate he was. I was astonished that for the first time, someone else validated what I had been living with my entire life. It wasn't just a secret fear or an unspoken anxiety anymore. Mark had seen it, seen him, and in so doing, had seen me.

CHAPTER TWELVE

My father's unhealthy influence became an issue in my relationship with Mark after a short while. We enjoyed a satisfying and eager sex life but I couldn't understand why, when I wanted to, I could not seduce him. My father had taught me that all men wanted sex all the time, and all women held the power by giving it to them, or not. But when other things were going on, Mark didn't look at me that way. Every time I took my clothes off, he didn't get excited and initiate sex. I felt unattractive and impotent. I complained about it and Mark thought it somewhat ridiculous. But I couldn't shake the feeling that I somehow lacked the enormous sexual power God gave to women. Was it my birthmark? My inexperience? Was something wrong with him? Why didn't he want sex all the time? This was just the beginning of a long, long journey that held me in its grip for many years.

So I kept James around. And he constantly filled me with that sense of power that was my birthright. I liked it, I needed it, and I wanted it. I just didn't want to act on it. One day James visited me at my apartment and noticed Mark's shoes by the door. He kept commenting on how big they were, which was odd because for such a tall man, he had average-sized feet. James was obviously agitated that I had any man's shoes in my place as it suggested the kind of intimacy I refused with him. Mark met him one day and made it clear that James was not a safe friend for me, much later calling him a sexual predator. It just wasn't his style to be jealous or expect any particular response on my part. It was that quality in Mark that allowed me to sift through these enormous issues in my own time and way. His self-confidence and patience were astounding. My father didn't even know men like Mark existed and he wouldn't have believed it if I had told him. And I never did.

My father came to visit and insisted on staying with me. By this time, my roommate had moved on and I was living alone, although Mark and I were spending most of our time at his apartment. I was completely traumatized at the thought of spending the night alone with my dad in my small apartment. When he first arrived and with that familiar grin on his face, he prodded me as to the extent of my sexual relationship with Mark, his version of a father-daughter talk. He let me know that while my mother should not know about it and would not approve, he did, and it would be our secret. He then asked if I was having regular orgasms, a subject so obviously fascinating to him that the conversation took place while waiting for his baggage to came up. I used that opening to tell him that I would be spending the night at Mark's apartment, as I usually did, during his visit. It was odd witnessing his excitement over my new sexual activity while at the same time observing his disappointment that I would not be staying with him alone overnight in my apartment. I honestly couldn't tell which was more important to him. I imagined his pride in my sexual awakening was similar to what other fathers would feel when their daughters made the honor roll or got a big promotion at work.

The next time I went to visit my parents in Bedford, Massachusetts, my father wandered the upstairs hallway between my room and theirs in search of birth control from the bathroom cabinet. In the dark, I could see his shadowy image preparing for their nightly sex ritual, fully excited. He made sure I could see. Mark wrote me letters while I was there.

Are you aware of all the subtle little things you do that belie your previous virginal status? They are all very appealing, by the way. What I'm getting at is that I love you and everything about you. What I'm thinking of especially is your letter. You've never had the opportunity to write down on paper and express your sexual desire before. I'm just guessing that you considered it but hesitated because of the newness and strangeness of expressing something so intimate and immediate by way of a letter which is so remote. I could be wrong, but believe me, kid, if you do feel a little silly, you sure don't have to write it down, I already know it. I just like to do it for you sometimes. I wish we were together.

CHAPTER THIRTEEN

Life settled in with Mark. We were both near completion of our college careers. I was working at the Dash Inn and saving every dime to go to New York after graduation, a plan that was in place before I met Mark. My Saturday shifts were long, starting at 5 pm and lasting until well after midnight. On a good, busy night, I left with a twenty dollar bill. One night after my shift, Mark and I were listening to *Rubber Soul* in his apartment. I was singing along and dancing on the coffee table. Suddenly I was overcome with the memory of listening to those same songs with my sister each night before we fell asleep at the apartment in Virginia where we stayed when we first arrived home from Turkey. I burst into tears and couldn't control the flood of emotion that the memory evoked. My sadness was overwhelming and still, its origin was completely unknown to me.

I dreaded the thought of leaving Mark behind but stuck to my plan to at least spend the summer following graduation in New York City. It became increasingly clear that Mark had no particular interest in practicing law. The bar exam was a grueling two and a half day experience after which he told me that if he did not pass, he would not be retaking the test. On the day the results were made available, he was first told that he had failed when his name could not be found on the list. It was a long twenty minutes or so after he came down to my apartment to announce he would never practice law before they called him back to say they had located his name after all, having originally looked for the second word in his last name rather than the first. It didn't matter much anyway as it turned out. He hated being a lawyer, delayed getting into it, and got out of it as fast as he could.

So off I went to the big city where I stayed at the proper Barbizon Hotel for Women. My college roommate was there with me for a while and we shared a room over the subway causing our beds to shake every time a train came by. I took dance class every day, sometimes more than one. The first week I was so sore I could hardly walk up and down the subway stairs. None of the studios were air conditioned and in the summer heat, it was easy to get in shape in a big hurry. I went to several calls for Broadway shows but couldn't really get excited over the auditions, afraid that I might be offered a contract for a year performing the same show eight times a week in a city I really didn't like. It was almost impossible being separated from Mark and I lived for his letters.

> *I'm lonesome. I miss you. I miss your warm nakedness next to me at night. Your face when I open my eyes and find you watching me. Has it been so very long? A departure so short the days are counted in hours. Questions left unanswered and solved by miles and time. And here I am and where are you? Beyond my touch, within my heart. This letter is a poem for you.*

When I could justify that I had been there long enough to fulfill my dream, I came home and ran straight into the arms of my future and never left again. There were plenty of times that I felt sexual electricity with another man that I would quietly and superficially explore but never act on. These men were attracted to me and even though I was not interested in a relationship with any of them, once they responded to me in that sexual way, I was hooked into the feeling of power it gave me. And those feelings and the way I acted on them gave me a strong connection to my father and the values with which he raised my sister and me. It had an addictive feeling to it, one that was hard to give up. While Mark was attracted to me in that way, he did not place sex in a category that had more importance than the desire to eat or sleep. It was just that quality that made him so right for me while also being the quality that I often resented and rebelled against. When I allowed that sexually tinged interaction with other men, it was to prove to myself that I could have that impact on a man, that I was not a defective woman as I so often believed myself to be. And I had to keep proving it. That need was in my DNA, my father's gift.

These seemingly harmless dalliances with other men were not in the same league as my relationship with James. We had lost touch now that I was no longer a student at the University. I missed the hit I got from the way he looked at me, the satisfaction of knowing how much he wanted me, how sensual and powerful it made me feel. I knew that no matter where he was or what he was doing, he would never be satisfied because I had resisted him and he would still be thinking about me and what was yet to be. It was the power of his desire that would someday bring him back to me.

CHAPTER FOURTEEN

Mark continued to resist lawyering and occasionally took work as a substitute teacher. I tried normal jobs, including an employment counselor position with an agency that required me to work under a pseudonym. That was the only part of the job that appealed to me. Then there was a management position at a Mormon owned bank that did not support women in executive roles. After I successfully represented the bank in a speech contest and was offered a promotion, I quit when turned down for a raise at my next review. We lived very cheaply in a small guest house behind the home of the contractor I used to date in college. We raised a litter of kittens deposited by the house cat, the calico Sally, and adopted one of her girls, Bugsy.

The public defender's office offered Mark a job, and he accepted. We bought a brand new townhouse together and I opened a dance studio in the small retail center within our planned lake community, for which my father served as executive director of the community association. My parents were thrilled to begin their retired life in a brand new home with a swimming pool on a golf course and a beautiful view of the sunset over the mountains. We spent many weekends at their house, swimming, playing "Hearts" and barbecuing. My father seemed proud that Mark and I did not feel the need to marry, with an "atta girl" tone to his support of our modern choice, tinged with a bit of jealousy at the relaxed standards we enjoyed. My mother would have greatly preferred matrimony, but was so enjoying our social relationship that she did not push. I wore an ERA bracelet. Some of the parents of my young dance students noticed my status as an unmarried woman living with a man right there in the neighborhood. That didn't bother me at all. What did bother me was that we were becoming careless about our use of birth control and I wanted to draw the line at becoming pregnant while still single. It was my suggestion that we get married, quickly and quietly, and stop using birth control altogether. After four years of living together, and immediately following the famous 1976 Suns-Celtics triple overtime playoff game, we announced to my parents that we would marry right away. My mother tried to arrange a nice, small Catholic wedding but the Church would not allow it since we were not active Catholics. She settled for arranging a party instead. With my parents and Mark's sister as witnesses, we were married at the Justice of the Peace on a Friday after work followed by Mexican food at our favorite place. Mark's father kindly sent us a check for one hundred dollars as a wedding gift and his mother completely ignored the occasion, persistently disapproving of our sinful living arrangement. We went home to our townhouse and nothing changed except I would begin to use the phrase "my husband" in conversation occasionally. I kept my maiden name, my father's name.

CHAPTER FIFTEEN

I added eight pounds to my ninety-five pound frame seemingly overnight. Pregnancy agreed with me and I continued to teach dance as my body ballooned. I felt very sexual throughout but it didn't seem to affect Mark that way. My very pregnant body outfitted in tangerine colored sheer lingerie did not lure him to the bedroom as I carefully planned one evening. I was crushed, left to feel unattractive, unfeminine, humiliated and miserable. Nothing was more devastating to me than when Mark rejected my occasional sexual advances, a constant reminder of my failure as my father's daughter.

Huge, sunburned and tired of waiting, I ignored my doctor's advice to eat light because the birth was eminent. We went to a movie and then out for a chimichanga with everything. In the middle of the night, I told Mark I was in labor and it was time to go to the hospital. He did not believe me, having endured more than one false alarm in the past few weeks, and suggested I go back to bed. I insisted on going right away and he called my parents who met us there. The doctor had been right about eating light and I sincerely regretted the big Mexican meal. Labor was natural and productive until we got into the delivery room. The doctor had estimated the baby to be around seven pounds but said anything over eight pounds would require a Caesarian section due to my small size. Having no luck pushing, it was decided that I would be put to sleep for a few moments for a long forceps delivery. Mark was allowed to stay, having already proven his Dutch stoicism throughout, even though it was strictly against the rules once the mother was put under. I awoke to see my husband holding our strapping baby boy, screaming at the top of his lungs, fists clinched. At eight pounds, six ounces, the doctor had misjudged his birth weight. My parents greeted me in the hall as I was wheeled out to a recovery room where I was left alone while the nurse took the baby to be cleaned up and weighed. Mark and my parents followed the baby. Those were the loneliest few moments of my life.

My father staked a claim on our boy, Andrew, from the very start. He was the male child my father had longed for and he had big dreams for him. It was obvious that he intended to influence our son's life in as many ways as he could, molding him in his own image. On the day of my studio's annual dance recital, my father planned to take Andrew to see Santa Claus before bringing him to the performance. Andrew was so excited that he ran full speed for the door, tripped on the sharp edge of an ottoman, and opened a cut on his eyebrow. My father took him to the emergency room to be stitched up and then brought Andrew to the show with a fresh scar and arms reaching out for his mommy.

During this time, my mother became agitated over my father's behavior and developed suspicions as to his fidelity. It wasn't the first time she had worried about the possibility that he was cheating on her but she seemed to be more concerned than usual. She found receipts in his pockets that fueled her suspicions and as always, said that if she found out he was being unfaithful to her, she would leave him. I also noticed his erratic behavior. He called me at home from time to time in strange, often bizarre moods, once saying he was considering suicide. He told me that men were imprisoned for the kinds of things he had thought about and done. I had to seclude myself while breast feeding Andrew due to my father's unnatural and certainly unfatherly interest in watching. He had developed a relationship with a young woman at work that my mother found upsetting, worried that she might be the other woman. My mother continued inappropriately confiding in me about their sex life. She spoke of how they had sex very regularly, often nightly, and how lucky they were to so often climax simultaneously. This served only to make me feel uncomfortable and depressed, emphasizing my husband's lack of consuming interest in sex with me, not to mention how disturbing it was to visualize their intimate habits in my already intensely screwed up mind. It even set up a sort of competition that, in this area, I was destined to lose.

CHAPTER SIXTEEN

My sister now had two children. She had found religion, hosting Bible meetings at her home and attending church. Since we were not close physically or emotionally, it was hard for me to fathom this change in her. When she came to visit, I couldn't wait to share a new album by Patti Smith that had captured my attention. The first track began with Patti's irreverent, throaty voice singing "Jesus died for somebody's sins, but not mine." That was all it took for Kathy to tell me that she didn't like the song and to please turn it off. This was not the sister I knew at all, bright and educated with a social curiosity and an open mind. It was clear she was searching for answers but I thought it highly unlikely she would find them in a Southern church. I didn't know the questions yet and wondered if she did either.

I was pregnant again, happily so, and Mark and I began to feel very uncomfortable around my parents. Their marriage seemed to be taking a disturbing turn and we were having trouble distancing ourselves and our family from the fallout. Mark was unhappy as a public defender and I was ready to give up my dance studio, already knowing it was not nearly satisfying enough to be a permanent career for me. Mark and I went to the movies one afternoon during my fat, unattractive pregnancy phase. I was devastated to run into James and his wife there, knowing for certain that whatever hope I had that he was still interested in me was shattered now that he had seen me in such a state. With money Grandlady gave me, we bought a home in Colorado where it was our intention to birth our second child, take a break from working for a while and concentrate on our young family. I sold my studio, Mark resigned from his job, we sold our home and said goodbye to my parents. Soon after we arrived, on a stormy night in early October, our son Peter was born, the child I believed was a girl until the moment I laid eyes on him. Instead he was an intuitive, sensitive boy. Andrew prepared for Peter's homecoming by putting some of his favorite toys in the bassinet next to the sunny dining room window.

One quiet afternoon, I was watching Oprah Winfrey. She had recently come out as a sexual abuse survivor and was hosting a show on the subject. Having had the luxury of being away from my father for a while, I felt more able to reflect on my parents and the dark, confusing issues that seemed to run just below the surface of our lives. Oprah captured my full attention as she educated the audience as to the scope of sexual abuse which was not limited to actually being raped as many presumed. She gently taught that whenever a girl or a woman felt violated by an inappropriate touch or even just being treated in a sexual manner, no matter the severity, it could have the same effect. She discussed the issue of broken trust when the sexual abuse occurs within a family unit, of the secrecy, the control, the power and the emotional devastation that follows. It was as though I suddenly stood up inside myself and instantly recognized the feelings that had swirled in me for so very long. I realized my father was a classic sexual abuser and even though he had never actually raped me, he had molested me, and probably my sister, and had raised us in a sexually charged environment. It was frightening but also thrilling to achieve this sudden clarity and although it ultimately led to dramatic and complex problems that I could not yet even imagine, I will always be grateful to Oprah for opening this window to me. The light came streaming in and I was fully energized to get to the business of explaining everything to my parents and my sister now that I understood it so we could all face the truth and heal as a family. Little did I know that such healing would never occur even though I would spend the next twenty years of my life dedicated to the mere possibility.

I immediately wrote to my father and told him that he had sexually abused me, citing specific examples and years of feelings caused by his inappropriate behavior. He put the letter away in a drawer, did not share its contents with my mother, and did not respond. I also called my sister right away, spilling out my new understanding of our father, barely taking a breath, assuming that this revelation would provide relief to her as well. It became clear right away that this was no revelation to her and she seemed devastated that her secret, their secret, had been uncovered. She did not wish to discuss it and became anxious, depressed and withdrawn. Her marriage was failing and would soon end, and she had become increasingly promiscuous with a growing alcohol problem. I didn't know enough at the time to understand that she was sinking into classic sexual abuse victim behavior. I was still trying to figure out the scope and impact of the truth about my father and its effect on my own life. Remembering that when I was molested by my father, I did nothing and told no one made it easier for me to understand why my sister had kept her dreadful secret for so many years and why she was still so unprepared and unwilling to speak about it.

CHAPTER SEVENTEEN

Our superficially idyllic life in Colorado came to an end when we ran out of money. The only place we could go was back to Arizona where Mark was a member of the state bar and I had enough contacts to find work. We stayed with my parents for a while as we tried to rebuild our lives. My father was in bad, if not worse, shape than when we had left. I remember him coming into the living room in front of my mother, Mark and me wearing nothing but tight, white underwear, showing us a rash all over his body. This incident exemplified the deteriorating situation with my parents. That my father would parade around in front of us in only his underwear literally showing off a rash seemed both completely natural and terribly revolting. I tried to imagine Mark's father, a dignified Dutch physician, doing such a thing. My father drank and we were certain that he was also abusing prescription drugs such as Valium. He seemed headed for a breakdown as my mother became more and more agitated, with me as her reluctant confidant.

Mark took a job as an attorney that he hated and I was able to land a few paying jobs choreographing musicals and operas. We rented a home in the same community where we had previously lived. My father had been hired away and was now running a similar lake community a few miles away. My sister was planning to marry again, a doctor with a cocaine addiction, reflecting her own out of control lifestyle. She begged me to come to the wedding but I refused, urging her to reconsider her decision. Their short, stormy marriage that included physical abuse ended with her life spiraling out of control and her ex-husband entering in-house rehabilitation. I was able to convince her to relinquish custody of her kids to their father in Alabama, now remarried.

We were struggling financially and my father was planning to open a management company using the experience he had gained running planned communities since his Air Force retirement. He begged me to join him, stating that I had not used my brain to its potential while being so involved in the arts. It was this connection he had made between us my whole life, that we were both smart people, that formed the only positive bond we ever really had and it was tempting. He said that we could make nice jobs for ourselves, be our own bosses, and one day I would have the freedom to pursue my artistic career without having to worry about money. I agreed to work part-time for him and continue my arts work at the same time. My mother would also help out at the office. Mark had already lost his attorney job and I knew he would never have another. He agreed to stay home with the boys while I tried out the new business venture with my father. The strain of a new business start-up along with teaching dance and choreographing shows on nights and weekends was much more than I expected. The combined hours were brutal. But I thoroughly enjoyed working on the musicals at the University and cast the boys in them from time to time. Andrew had a small featured part as a cabin boy in *HMS Pinafore* and both boys appeared in a national award winning opera, one playing a snail and the other a dancing cricket. I used my dance students as angels in a beautiful production of *Hansel and Gretel*.

My father continued to lure me with the notion that I would

have regular business hours for the first time in my life and would be able to spend my evenings and weekends with Mark and the boys. So I joined the company full-time at a salary of $5 per hour. We tripled our gross each year for the first three years and rapidly built a successful, diverse management company. I continued to teach dance.

I had a young woman in my class whose name sounded familiar to me. I asked if she was related to a man I knew of the same last name. She said yes, that my James was her father. She was the little girl in the family photo I had first seen at the townhouse pool over ten years ago that James had hoped I would never see. She must have told her dad about my inquiry so he made it a point to pick her up from class one evening. He stuck his head in the door to say hello. I looked good that night, in great shape, dressed in leotard and tights, quite different from that pregnant day at the movies a few years before. He left with a buzz on, promising to assist me with my latest work, an arts project about the Vietnam War. He had an impressive position at the University and would introduce me to various high school principals he knew so we could present the educational work in the classroom. It gave us a reason to be in touch, to get together.

Our first meeting was for lunch where it was quickly concluded that absolutely nothing had changed over the years we had been apart. We stood out in the parking lot as we parted. I was wearing a navy and white vertical striped silk blouse tucked into a short, straight navy linen skirt with hose and heels. He reached over to brush my long hair from my face when the wind blew and his hand slipped across my breast.

As if things were slowly moving into place for the perfect storm, Michael also reappeared in my life. We took the boys to Washington DC for a holiday, and he met us for a short visit in a beautiful park.

That marked the beginning of our renewed friendship. He had not changed; he was quiet and thoughtful, incredibly intuitive, and still in love with me. He worked for the Smithsonian Museum of American Art and had become a fine painter himself. He shared a studio with other artists in an old warehouse in the District. When I returned home, we began to communicate from time to time by phone. He would listen for hours as my personal situation slowly became more emotionally dangerous and stressful. We were developing a mature, adult version of our innocent high school relationship.

CHAPTER EIGHTEEN

Looking back, it is hard to imagine how I could have moved back to the desert and allowed my parents to have such a strong role in our lives. They saw the boys frequently and knowing my father's history, I assumed that because they were male children, they would be safe. We would sometimes put them to bed at my parents' home while we would eat a late dinner and I noticed that my father would go "lay with them" when they wouldn't settle down. I had a serious talk with him and told him we were not comfortable with that, asking him to not only stop going into their room after they had been put down, but also forbidding him to discuss anything of a sexual nature with them at any time or at any age. He agreed. This was representative of that time when our family secret was somewhat acknowledged because I had insisted but in a quiet, non-threatening way. It was my period of continuing denial.

One evening I noticed he was not with us in the family room and walked down the hall to the boys' room and found the door cracked and my father in with them. I heard him speaking to them in a way that I believed was inappropriate and became very upset. How could I have ever believed that we could trust him by simply keeping a close eye on him? Even catching him in an inappropriate situation with my kids did not change things. I later learned that when they spent the night, he would come in to "lay" with them in only his tight, white underwear that the boys called "tightie whities." Peter always hoped that Papa would not choose his bed but when he did, he would hug the wall desperately trying to avoid physical contact with his grandfather. Andrew watched adult entertainment on cable television in my parents' bedroom. Occasionally his grandmother would come in and say that he shouldn't be watching that, but then left without making sure that he turned it off.   They were routinely exposed to situations and references with sexual overtones.

My sister moved to Phoenix to start a new life and even though she didn't have custody of her children, they would come to visit. Kathy's sales job at an upscale hotel required travel so my parents would often care for her kids while she was away. My mother had a gleeful grin on her face when she spoke of how she had found Kathy's daughter watching television, stimulating herself sexually. And again when describing how her grandson had become sexually aroused when she showed him how good a piece of satin lingerie felt against his skin. It was the same grin my father wore when telling us about the facts of life, and enjoying our Playboy playmates game in the tub. That is when I began to understand that my mother was as serious a threat as my father. She had been thoroughly indoctrinated into his value system and had accepted it as her own. It was all she knew.

I continued to lobby for facing the truth as a family, connecting my sister's growing troubles to the abuse, pointing out the problems to my mother, and continually confronting my father. It permeated our work life together at the company as well as our social life away from the office. The more I pushed for open acknowledgement of our problems, the more they resisted and the worse things got. My mother argued that if my sister were the primary victim, why did she not make these claims and why was she still on good terms with her father? My father closed the door to my office to quietly tell me that, yes, he had been inappropriate with Kathy but only because he was trying to educate her as to the ways of the "Playboy generation." He in no way acknowledged that it had anything to do with her problems. I later read that his "I was educating her" excuse ranks second on the list of most often stated reasons that fathers give for sexually abusing their daughters. It was comforting to know that he was textbook, nothing special.

I hired a young woman to work for me, very bright and very well endowed. My father was, of course, infatuated with her large breasts and despite her overtly religious nature, she enjoyed showing them off. She and I got along wonderfully. One Friday after work, we stayed after closing to move some furniture. We began speaking about our personal lives and she disclosed that she had been sexually abused by her grandfather. I told her our family story and she surprised me by saying she already knew simply by observing my father and the family dynamics she witnessed daily. She became a trusted confidant although from time to time our relationship was stormy and complex. She was entangled in a very destructive relationship with a priest who was also sexually abusing her, right under the nose of his wife and children with whom she spent a lot of time. He would visit her at work and I recognized the sexual obsession he had for her because I had seen it twice, in my father and in James. She fought to protect her need to be sexual with him even after I understood what was happening and encouraged her to step away. He had convinced her that God wanted them to be together. At the same time, I was slowly becoming overly involved with James, my version of the same thing. Her abuser, the priest, was also her counselor. I had no counselor, just my growing addiction to the sexual power of James and his attraction to me. And mine to him.

My sister continued to struggle and it became apparent that she felt she should also participate in this thriving business that my father and I had worked so hard to build. My father wouldn't hire her without my permission, respecting my position of authority, which I appreciated. After speaking at length with my sister, we all agreed we would give it a try. Shortly after she was installed in the small, boxy office with no windows between my father's and mother's offices, I was struck by how much it seemed like the tiny bedroom they had banished her to when we lived in Turkey. She felt it also and began to emotionally crumble. She acted out at work, made unreasonable demands, and as part of her duties, hired two men. One would later rape two women, including one of our managers, and then his own three-year-old daughter. He was given a long prison term. The other was an intensely intelligent, secretive, manipulative man who attempted to take control of the company behind my back. He was fired and went on to become an attorney after perjuring himself as a witness in a case against us. I disclosed it on his Arizona bar inquiry but it wasn't enough to keep him from being accepted. My sister became deeply depressed, often non-functional, and my parents feigned ignorance as to what could be troubling her. I kept pointing out the problem—sexual abuse—but my position remained completely unsupported. The psychologist who was consulted stated that if she was not huddled in a fetal position in bed for weeks on end, and could get up and get dressed and be somewhat productive, she did not require hospitalization. My parents clung to that and proclaimed her okay enough.

I continued to work at the company, continued to see and hear from James, and continued to press my extended family for acknowledgement of the real problem. All three stated that they were very sorry that I had ever uncovered the truth and liked it much better when it had been something we didn't discuss. They persisted in their desire to just move on and get things back to the way they used to be. But I couldn't do that. Instead, I kept sliding down my own slippery slope while at the same time, trying to save them. Occasionally I would write to them, trying a different approach to making them understand. Probably it was the relief I got from writing the words that really appealed to me.

Dear Mom and Dad,

I cannot bear another confrontation about Kathy, after having experienced one with each of you this week, so I thought maybe a letter would help.

We have all said repeatedly over the years that we wished and hoped that Kathy would seek therapy in order to understand herself better thereby improving the quality of her life. Dad was even instrumental in encouraging her to make that first important step with you, Mom, providing the name of a doctor. Now, rather miraculously in my eyes, she has really done it. And will be doing it for a long time, maybe even the rest of her life. I have repeatedly reported to you that she is doing well, making substantial progress and feeling 100% better about herself. Both she and her doctor have put a condition on this phase of her treatment requiring distance from the both of you. This was a professional decision based on his assessment of his patient and a personal one for Kathy. In my opinion, you have no choice but to honor that decision, not just by respecting it, but by supporting it and trying to understand it from your heart. Unselfishly.

There are certain dynamics of this family that you don't need to take responsibility for but need to acknowledge. There is certain symbolism in the situation with Kathy which can help us to understand those dynamics. Kathy's request for privacy certainly seems to represent her first attempt at taking control of her own life. Long overdue but never too late. Mother, in our talk in the car, you actually used the phrase that "Kathy has taken control of this situation" as though it were unacceptable for her to do so. Then you went on to say that she could make this choice personally but not professionally. When I explained that it was perfectly logical for Kathy to answer to me and indeed it was working well, you repeated that you had control over business and would not accept this indefinitely. I warned you not to use ownership of the business as a power tool to insist on her communication because at this point with Kathy, personal and business are one and the same. The symbolism here seems to be the use of the business as a "justifiable" means of control. There is no business reason at this time to insist on Kathy's direct and personal communication.

Friday morning, Dad, you came into my office soliciting my help stating that something had to break with Kathy. You however didn't bother to use the business "excuse", you simply stated that you and Mother, especially, couldn't handle it. You said Kathy was "dead" to you. More symbolism. Kathy is more alive in her own right now than ever before yet she's "dead" to you. Despite the fact that I assure you of her well-being. You went on to say that her doctor should change his approach to accommodate your feelings. This is an incredible statement to me. I had just stated how well they both thought the treatment was progressing. You are both completely immersed in how it is affecting you. The conclusion one might draw is that as your daughter, she is expected to put your welfare above hers and worse yet, feel pressure and guilt for her very healthy decision not to do so. I support her courage in this very difficult decision and will stand like a lion at her gate to insure her right to continue.

Dad, you went on to specifically state that she must write a letter to Mother saying that she loved her and was still her daughter. What value could you possibly gain from a letter that you demand saying what you want to hear? In my opinion, it is you two who should be writing her a letter stating total acceptance of her decision and letting her know that, although it is painful, she must take all the time she needs without worrying about you. She has enough to worry about to get herself well. You also stated that you two would be in the hospital if Kathy didn't stop this. Again, this would seem to place responsibility on Kathy for your state of mind. Just as Kathy is boldly taking responsibility for herself, you two must do the same. If you are having trouble coping, get your own help. You may learn something that will help us all cope.

If you desire to really begin the process of understanding how you find yourself in this spot, I am willing to participate in family counseling with the both of you. However, you must be willing to deal with truth and reality. I am not willing to go under any other circumstance. Kathy will not be willing to tolerate denial any longer.

These Kinney family problems are taking a toll on me personally as I try to support each of you. I don't know how much strength I have left for that and wish again you would find a professional to help you cope so that I might be relieved of that role.

It's been a real relief to say this today. I feel it's the first constructive thing I've done for myself in all of this.

CHAPTER NINETEEN

I arranged for Kathy to relocate to Tucson where she would run our satellite operation. Her condition spiraled out of control after she moved. Her drinking became habitual and problematic and she was leading a promiscuous, dangerous lifestyle. She could no longer function professionally and my mother was given the terrible task of terminating her employment. We ultimately gave her the entire Tucson operation to completely cut business ties. She formed a partnership with an employee, and somehow he ended up with one hundred percent ownership of the company, even sending over a tow truck in the middle of the night to take her company car. Having lost everything, she finally landed in 30-day in-house rehab where she was diagnosed with Post Traumatic Stress Disorder as a result of long-term sexual abuse. It was determined that her drinking and other addictive behaviors were symptomatic of the primary diagnosis of PTSD. My parents visited her there and attended the family activities. I did not. I couldn't bear to. The counselor interviewed my mother and father and later said that the father gave the most sanitized version of "the big one" that she had ever heard. Further, that the mother was in the most massive denial she had ever seen, describing what it was like sitting across the table from the mother and father, watching the mother smile angelically at the father as he explained that he was actually only trying to move my sister into sexual adulthood.

Kathy lost her home, continued drinking, and lived in a horrible halfway house for a long while, being unable to afford another place to live and unable to keep a job. I never visited her there either although once when in town for a professional conference drove by to see what it was like. The sight of that terrible place has stayed with me. How could a member of our family have come to this? My parents were unwilling to commit enough money month to month to insure that she would have a roof over her head. The uncertainty was devastating for her so I negotiated on her behalf an arrangement where my parents would pay rent each month for a small house and I would contribute half of that amount myself for expenses. Thus began a long period, ongoing today, where she would suffer deep depression and anxiety, would never want to leave her home, would gain close to one hundred pounds, would not be able to work, and would never give up her relationship with our parents. After every visit to their home, she would crash into a deep depression for weeks.

CHAPTER TWENTY

In the meantime, I continued to reconnect with Michael, writing him from time to time about my life. The letters were sweet and informal. He talked about his artwork and we made plans to attend our 20th high school reunion in Washington DC. He had hated high school and had no interest whatsoever in seeing our old pals, being reminded of times he considered painful. But I very much wanted him to go with me and used all my considerable influence with him to cajole him into saying yes.

But I had another agenda. Having been only barely sixteen when I graduated and not fully "formed" at the time, it was very important for me to go back and show my former classmates who I turned out to be and frankly, how I turned out to look after I had finally physically matured. On one of our family beach trips to California that summer, I found the perfect little black dress, little being the operative word. It was a short skirt with a close fitting top with three quarter sleeves and a scoop back. I was in great shape, my signature hair was long and wavy, and I was ready to be noticed. Michael was traumatized at the very thought of it all, but I insensitively insisted that he join me, refusing to take no for an answer.

I had taken a room at the hotel where the reunion was being held and he knocked on the door, slides of his artwork in hand. When I answered and he saw me in the black dress, I thought he was going to faint. That was pretty much the last I saw of him until he left later that evening. I am ashamed of how insensitive I was to his feelings and have asked his forgiveness many times. While checking in, one of our high school's football stars approached me and asked my name. I pointed to my name tag, which also had my senior photo on it. He said he didn't know me. I said we had been in class together. He said no, that wasn't possible. He would have definitely remembered me. *A good start*, I said to myself. Maybe it was because most of my former classmates still lived in the more conservative East, but they acted like they had never even seen an outfit like mine. It definitely had the desired effect and I was attracting a lot of attention. The lead singer in the band, a member of my sister's class, was dedicating songs to me and suggesting we get together later. I tried to keep an eye out for Michael, feeling guilty about abandoning him, but he had disappeared into the woodwork. I had attracted the attention of a guy who was quite intoxicated, someone I did not remember from school but Michael did, and not fondly. He kept a beat on me and it felt creepy and unsafe.

Finally, Michael said he was tired and intended to leave for home. I begged him to stay but to no avail. I walked him out to the hotel lobby, still glowing from my triumph. His gaze, the intensity of it, the way he knew me and completely understood what was happening to me that night, took me by surprise. I very suddenly saw him in a completely different way and it washed over me like a wave as he stood there inhabiting my feelings. He quietly took me in his arms to say goodbye. In that embrace was a deep and intense desire, not only him for me but me for him as well. I couldn't easily let go of him and my body was responsive in a way that completely contradicted the raw sexual urges that James provoked. This was a sexual feeling that I imagined to be healthy, based on love and affection, that would not be explosive or performance based nor would it be the comforting opposite of my father's sexual obsession. No, it would have been slow and long and intimate and quiet and artistic and sensitive and I thought of it as healing and good. I so longed for it that I could barely resist taking his hand and leading him to my room. For the first of many, many times to come, it was Michael who did the right thing, who exercised care and restraint for both of us, taking my arms from around his neck and refusing to allow me to walk him to his car. It was protective and sweet and caring but still remains one of the most powerful sexual moments I have ever experienced.

As I gathered myself and headed back to the party, the creepy man found me and began to follow me aggressively through the empty halls. I was scared, moving faster and faster. It was the only time in my life I felt like I barely escaped being raped. The next morning over breakfast, his wife began speaking to everyone about that bitch in the little black dress who was pursuing her husband, obviously not recognizing me from across the table. It was awkward to say the least. Never in my life had I been characterized in that way. At thirty-six years old, I was coming of age sexually through the long-term mentorship of my father, James' lust for me, and the love of this gentle man who seemed to protect me from it all. That night further complicated my already complicated situation. A delicate balance, Michael called it.

CHAPTER TWENTY-ONE

I returned home to pick up life where emotional betrayal began to feel more the norm than not. Otherwise things ran along. Actually, it was Mark who provided the delicate balance between me and insanity. He allowed. He made it all my decision. And then he validated, giving me full credit. He didn't see me just as a sensual creature, or just as anything, but instead as a woman, respecting and recognizing all my facets. He had no expectations of me. If I didn't want to have sex, it was my natural right and he respected that. The problem was that I always did, even when he didn't, and he expected the same consideration back. Respect and a high regard for personal freedom seemed to trump simply wanting sex. That high road seemed a little too high for me to reach on a regular basis. So whereas I perceived that most women detested the male inclination to sexually objectify women, I myself actually longed for it in a way. It was easy for James to provide that because he did not have to concern himself with any other aspects of my life, responding to me only as a sensual woman to be enjoyed from time to time. An unfair luxury and advantage for him. Sampling the golden nugget without having to go into the mine. But I felt I could not live without affecting a man in this way.

There was a tremendous amount of responsibility that came with the respect and support that my husband so freely gave to me. I wanted a career, so he not only supported it but agreed to stay home to give me the opportunity without sacrificing the well-being of our children. In that regard, I was a male with a wife at home. Men could be valued at home for the same things for which they were valued in their careers. Taking charge, making decisions, dictating timing, and being leaned on. Not exactly highly valued female qualities. When I was not at work, I did not wish to be all of the things I had to be when I was in charge of everything. So a complete change had to be made on the drive home. Back to a woman. Soft and nurturing, gentle and kind, wife and mother. Not so easy on just a five-minute drive.

James responded to the male part of me as a confident, successful professional, and he actually possessed certain qualities such as emotional vulnerability, which I thought of as deeply feminine. Being able to provoke and affect these feelings in him as compared to my stoic, strong, structured and stable husband was very appealing to me.

Our encounters affected James deeply. His demeanor would turn dark when things were particularly difficult or frustrating, and like me, it could make him physically ill. Once on a Saturday morning, knowing I was scheduled to be working at my office, he came by to see me even though I had told him that other workers would also be there. In a burst of emotion, he threw himself on his knees at my feet, hugging my legs, begging me to be with him. I gently pulled him away with my hands on his face, aware that someone could actually be observing this, amazed at his display of uncontrollable desire. When I walked him to his car, he reached his hand up under my shirt to feel my skin, then moved it down inside my jeans. He had a way of knowing when he could safely touch me, even when others were around, so they wouldn't know. Then he just drove away.

The effect this had on me was profound. Nothing else matched it. I entertained the idea that I should somehow take offense at these liberties, imagining that my husband would think I should take it as a sign of disrespect. But it was quite the opposite. He was the only man alive that I could allow to treat me this way and I was determined to have the feeling, no matter what. Why did people assume that only men had such intense sexual feelings and would do almost anything to satisfy their cravings such as cheating on their wives, or lying? I felt my need was as strong as any man's. Be the pilot, be the doctor, be anything you like.

It was shocking that I was able to so completely separate my secret life and growing sexual conflicts from my real life and I tried very hard, usually with some success, to forget that this was exactly how my father did it for so many years. It was also how James did it as well in his role of husband, father, and intimate to so many women. The more I engaged in the long extended ritual of foreplay with James, the more I had to rely on my contact with Michael. He had become my closest friend, my most trusted confidant. He worried over my behaviors, obviously escalating to what seemed the inevitable transgression with James, a transgression I believed I was destined to commit and that I knew in advance would ruin my life. And yet he did not try to convince me to stop. He just listened and offered unconditional love and support. He was hauntingly protective of me and I could feel his love literally embrace me.

I began to write in an effort to retain some type of control over feelings that were taking over my life.

I never feel well anymore. I doubt that I have a disease, at least not of the medically diagnosable type. Perhaps a social disease. A physical social disease.

My state of mind began affecting my health when I was ten years old. We were told we couldn't take our family dog with us to Turkey because Turks ate dogs and it wasn't safe. Pepe, our Pekinese, was actually my dog, a gift for my eighth birthday after a seriously choreographed campaign to convince my parents that I absolutely must have a dog. They surprised me by sending Pepe down the hall with a St. Patrick's Day green ribbon around his neck. I was so happy. He became my constant companion and slept with me every night. My parents sent him off to live with Grandlady in Florida as we left for language school in Washington DC before leaving for Turkey. I was completely devastated and literally mourned his absence. Having to leave my first boyfriend, Tommy Ognisty, behind as well made life unbearable. I developed mysterious and undiagnosable health problems. When Grandlady told us that Pepe couldn't stay because he was disturbing their parakeet who was nothing short of family, it was decided that we would take the chance and Pepe would accompany us to Turkey. I began to feel much better right away.

I'm not ten anymore but my illnesses are still undiagnosable. When I got the family business under control, the payoff was to be able to work on a creative Vietnam project that meant a lot to me. But I wore the collective grief of the Vietnam combat veterans like a tight sweater that just wouldn't quite fit over my head again once I had put it on. Still do. I began to feel tired, but not sick. I began having headaches. When we had to fire my sister from the family business, she faced for the first time that my father had indeed sexually abused her throughout her life with me being her only witness and support in this revelation. She stopped speaking to us and I became the focus of my parents' pain, expectations and future. My head is no longer the only thing that is aching. My muscles feel like bricks. I begin to dread going to the office. Now my headaches last for days and my stomach is involved, too. I look awful. I can't sleep because I have my episodes in the middle of the night when I have the time. Trying to diagnose the undiagnosable illness. I called my dear friend and nutritionist who has been the most successful in helping me deal with these things but he was too busy to talk to me. He suggested that he put his wife on the phone and we set up a phone appointment to discuss my symptoms in a few days. Wednesday at 10 alright? No fever, he said, so we can probably rule out the serious things. Take a hot shower and you'll feel better.

By now the energy has all gone and only the brain remains active. That really contributes to the undiagnosable nature of the problem. Worn out, beat down, you think about those people in Reader's Digest whose problems are much worse than yours and they have experienced a triumph of the human spirit. But their problems were so diagnosable, like cancer or being shot or paralyzed. It's cleaner somehow. Me, I just cry when I think about my sons' friends who have no childhood left at age twelve. Or my sister's emotional wounds that have left her in so much pain and so alone that she can barely function. And certainly my Vietnam vets who just keep going in spite of unimaginable grief and adversity. After age ten, I don't think it is quite so easy as getting your dog back to make it all better. Instead, just surviving the physical social disease seems an admirable goal. I don't know exactly how to do that, do you?

But as I sit here at my computer, it's now 2 am and the open window allows a very cool breeze to refresh me, which is a blessing at any time in the desert in May. My two boys and my husband are sleeping soundly and don't seem to miss me at the moment. And tomorrow I will feel well enough to go to the Little League game. My husband will be coaching, my older boy will coach third base, and my young son (who is still a child) will probably pitch and get a couple hits. I will watch with Zak's dad as we anguish over how the coach could leave that kid in with the bases loaded and no outs! Doesn't he want to win the game? We'll get home in time to watch the Phoenix Suns try to upset the best team in basketball during game five of the play-offs which have the entire community on fire. Of course, my older son is for the opposing team. If the home team wins, the younger son will stay wide awake and beg to watch the ten o'clock sports report in our room, too excited to sleep. If we lose, he may fall asleep early and the older son will want to watch the sports in our room so he can gloat over his victory. Either way. . .

My father did his part in my continuing education by promoting his disturbed philosophy on everything from current events to his perceived expertise on human behavior. One day while we were watching Peter compete in a tennis tournament, he proclaimed that there was "no such thing as rape." All women wanted it, he said. In that way, there was always consent. Even I had the belief that rape victims were chosen by their attackers for their highly valued sexual attractiveness, a quality that I feared I was missing. He and my mother thrived on the Anita Hill-Clarence Thomas hearings, repeatedly vilifying the woman who made those "ridiculous accusations against the judge who was, after all, just being a man." They were ecstatic when she was put in her place where she belonged and the judge was narrowly confirmed to the Supreme Court. My father used the Navy Tailhook scandal to justify his own behaviors with his "fighter pilots will be fighter pilots" philosophy. "See," he said to me, "that's just the way we are. No big deal. I'm no different from them." I tried to make the distinction that while those pilots may be disrespectful to military women, it is unlikely that their chauvinistic attitudes of entitlement extended to sexual behavior with their daughters. And then his theory that the sharp rise in breast cancer cases obviously reflected womens' continuing desire to be more like men. I don't know exactly what his secret life involved at that time, but I am certain that his many theories justified and validated all of it. He was at the top of his game.

CHAPTER TWENTY-TWO

With my sister now out of the work picture, my parents continued to exercise their financial control over the company as co-owners, not once offering me stock or an ownership role despite my significant and growing responsibility. Feeling confident that I had learned enough to run things, my father walked out the door one day and it seemed as though he was never coming back. His primary interest was the monthly profit/loss statement. My mother loved her role though and especially getting dressed to come in to work every day. She wasn't experienced or educated enough to actually hold a position of real responsibility but she reveled in the power of her ownership role. I was still an employee, stuck between the growing number of non-family employees and the owners, responsible for virtually everything. I knew it would be necessary for me to patiently run things until my father had grown completely comfortable playing golf and enjoying partial retirement. Then he would never want to come back, maybe wouldn't even be able to.

In the meantime, I planned to make a few demands. Preparing well in advance, I drove to their home for the meeting I requested, all of us agreeing that no more volatile family meetings should be held within earshot of the employees. I pumped up the volume on the stereo and found a driving rhythm track to which I chanted power, power, power, power, control, control, control, control, over and over again until I arrived in their driveway. I didn't want to show any sign of weakness and I wanted to begin to build my power base for the future. My demands were to be named the president; to take over my father's old office which was the largest in the complex; to have my own company credit card; to have a significant pay increase; and to have my father host a company-wide meeting for the purpose of announcing my promotion and corresponding authority. My parents met my demands, all the while nervously explaining that they were going to do these things on their own anyway. I had just beat them to it. I felt I had won my first battle but had no idea that the war would involve so much more than control of the company.

CHAPTER TWENTY-THREE

I met with James when I could and held him off the best I could. My ongoing writing reflected what was happening, the very act providing relief and occasionally a glimpse into the meaning of my behaviors, which now seemed to be growing more out of control. Because what I was doing seemed so unbearable in the light of day, in the light of my love for my family, in light of my own view of who I was, I wrote in third person, further underscoring my emotional detachment from this thing I did not believe myself to be capable of doing.

> *Sometimes she would go to his office. Maybe once they would just sit across the desk and chat innocently, trying to concentrate, smoldering underneath. Other times, depending on his mood, he would close the door, hold her, and run his hands over her small body. She loved his hands, curious and demanding, but always gentle and sensitive. He noticed everything, what she wore, how she sat, filling her with the strongest sense of herself that she had ever known. After she would leave, he would call later and say that his whole office was still full of her, still smelled like her. Sometimes on the phone, he would ask her what she was wearing, where she was sitting, and then tell her what he was thinking. Other times he was so tired of their lack of contact and privacy, he would just withdraw.*
>
> *He gave her his total attention, overwhelming her with romantic friendship and affection, listening and holding her hand as she*

gradually began to open up and depend on him. He still teased her with jokes of what he really wanted to do, but no pressure. She was consumed with him and his presence every moment of every day and spent tremendous energy just exercising her will to stay in control when every instinct in her said it was time to lose every ounce of control she had. Her head always stopped her. His approach was brilliant and patient. They met many times in various places. He admitted that he thought of her more than he should but assured her that even though he had come to love her, he was not in love with her. She had no idea how or what she felt but she listened to every thing he said and it began to get through, to absorb into her.

Once during what felt like an especially intimate lunch, he admitted that he was now in love with her. She hugged him that day as they were leaving and reached up to kiss him lightly on the lips. And so she started it. He talked about the kiss later, how he felt it all the way to his stomach. He always did that. The smallest, most wonderful things would occur between them and then he would bring them up, letting her know that he felt them and thought about them. This thrilled her.

When her family was out of town, she found herself agreeing to meet him one evening where she was planning to dine alone. She had decided on that occasion to let him close. She chose to walk from home. He arrived, wearing jeans, a lavender button down shirt with the sleeves perfectly rolled up, and cowboy boots. He joined her at her table and she was flushed at the sight of him. He had already eaten at the reception, which was his alibi for being with her. He said he would prefer to watch her eat anyway, that he loved to watch her eat. On the way out, she tried to talk him into playing golf with her over the next few days, a safe way to spend several hours together. He refused, saying that was not what he wanted. He explained that he cared deeply for her, cared about every breath she took. He said that. She faced his car, leaning against the door, totally lost as to what she should agree to. He came up behind her, covering her back with his chest. She could feel him breathe and the heat of his body against her, his face on her shoulder burying into her neck. Someone came out of the restaurant, looking over at them. He stepped away. When she turned around, her look drew him close again. She closed her eyes and lifted her face to him, knowing that he would know exactly what she wanted. For the first time really, he kissed her. And this was exactly what she wanted. She responded, starting slowly, allowing his tongue to roam, opening her mouth so that he could kiss her more deeply. They stopped, gazing at each other with such wonderful relief, and kissed again. She kissed first his top lip, then moved down, nipping at his lower lip. His lips were so full and rich, she felt that she could linger on them for hours. His hands moved to her breasts, gently and sweetly. They continue to kiss, now with more urgency. He was carried away. He whispered in her ear that he didn't think he could stop.

This snapped her back to reality and the present situation and she knew that this was as far as she could go this time. She insisted on walking home, he insisted on taking her in his car. She wouldn't let him, knowing that he would come in her empty house and they would be alone in there forever. He was unhappy but happy. He drove off to the lake after that, he later said. She always wished she had gone with him. She should have gone with him, wherever he went.

She did not feel the pavement under her feet walking home, following the moon. She stopped on the bridge, felt the breeze on her skin, floating. When she got home, she put on her satin nightie, sang and danced, touched herself and fell happily asleep.

The very next morning at work, my father took one look at me and said, "What happened to you?" It was as if he had witnessed my sex-charged encounter with James the night before, that familiar "playboy" grin on his face. The sex I hadn't yet had but that he seemed to be urging me to have in his secretive, all knowing "just between you and me" way. Yes, he knew. My God, he knew by looking at me.

CHAPTER TWENTY-FOUR

My parents' marriage continued to unravel as my mother's suspicions about my father's behavior continued to grow. She demanded that they seek counseling together. She chose the same therapist that had treated my sister. He was a tall, handsome man who really seemed to like my mother and she was drawn to him somehow, as a protector. My father didn't really care who they saw because he assumed that any therapist could be manipulated and outsmarted. It wasn't like he was actually planning to change his life or heal his marriage or succumb to our ongoing need for acknowledgement of his sexual misconduct with us. He would just endure the experience until my mother got it out of her system. But something happened in those sessions and one day it all blew up. My mother was very upset and isolated herself for a while, choosing only to tell me that he had admitted infidelity. Her humiliation at actually learning what she already knew overpowered her desire to tell me everything about his numerous indiscretions. Despite her years of proclaiming that she would leave upon confirmation of being cheated on, it didn't take her that long to decide that she would forgive him and rebuild their marriage because, after all, she loved him. How disappointing that was to me as I still held out hope that one day she would recognize him for who he was and rush to our side, profusely apologizing for doubting her daughters' stories, and assuring us that she believed us and would always take our side. I saw his admission in therapy as a real opportunity for her to change sides. But she didn't. Things worsened as she became his champion in forgiveness and understanding. And of more consequence, that moment of weakness, of letting his guard down, of revealing himself, caused an immediate power shift in their marriage. Now she had the upper hand knowing what she knew and her forgiveness sealed his fate. He would stay with her, he would eventually convert to Catholicism as she had always wanted and he would try to go along with her carefully constructed view of a marriage saved by love. He had been neutered by his own hand.

My mother never told me the details of his disclosure in therapy that day. But my sister claimed to know the details directly from my father. They still shared a kind of perverse intimacy, honed over years of practice, that you could see at a party when they would put their heads close together, drinks in hand, and whisper to one another. He enjoyed sharing his secrets with her, those that he never talked to me or my mother about. My sister reported that there were numerous affairs over the years, including the woman with whom he was living while serving in Southeast Asia, along with an eight-year affair since they had retired in Phoenix. She said that he had confided a recurring dream in which he was knee deep in "shit." My sister also told me that she was certain he was sleeping with our maid in Germany and that she had once walked in on him and Grandlady in a compromising position during one of her visits. My mother put a nice bow on everything and proceeded as if it was all worked out.

I encouraged my sister to talk to my mother and reveal more detail about the sexual abuse, details that my mother could not possibly deny as part of my continuing, relentless effort to initiate family healing. My father was going out of town for a few days and my mother invited both of us over for a girls' only visit. We sat with my mother in her living room while my sister gathered up all the courage she could summon. She stated that our father had been sexually inappropriate with her most of her life. My mother dismissed it at first, then challenged her to prove it, to give more detail, to say exactly what she meant. Once again, I had to encourage my sister to continue. She chose a story that happened in Turkey, the place where the most intense abuse took place. She asked our mother to recall the trip my father took to Paris. He brought us each white French jeans and colorful, stretchy tank tops. But she said my father also brought her a present that only they knew about. It was a pair of crotchless French panties. I will never forget the look that passed over my mother's face upon hearing this dreadful revelation. It was as if the information went in one ear before being slowly and meticulously processed in her head on the way to her voice. She paused for a long while, then said that it would have been impossible for my sister to have had an item of clothing that she, as her mother, would not have seen or known about. After all, she did the laundry and had access to her bedroom and her drawers. Where, she demanded to know, did she keep these panties? My sister said that obviously they were hidden so as not to be found. My mother repeated her demand to know where, where could she have hidden them? If they existed, she would have seen them somewhere. It was so disturbing to be present for this scene, for this complete betrayal of a mother's solemn duty to protect, or even just believe, her child, that I left the house immediately. It was hard to leave my sister there, but although she was crushed and emotionally devastated by my mother's cruel response to her painful disclosure, she still refused to leave. She always took it, from both of my parents. She had been raised to put their needs first. But I couldn't, not on that day, and increasingly not on any day.

A few days later, I spoke to my mother about her abhorrent behavior, stating that she should confront my father and see what he had to say about Kathy's claim. She said she already had. I asked how he responded. She said, "Well, he didn't deny it. What does that tell you?" I said it told me it was true. She didn't argue. But that was the end of it. She never pursued it after that, never apologized to my sister, never spoke of it again. The literal face of angry denial on my mother that day is one of the ugliest sights I have ever seen.

Tired of hearing that "nothing happened to me" so why was I the one who was making such a big deal of all of this when Kathy was supposedly the real victim, I finally told my mother about how my father had molested me on the eve of my sister's wedding. Taken aback, she said that she would ask him about it, possessing no other answer at that moment. She came back to me later and announced that she had indeed spoken to her husband about my claim. Yes, he remembered the incident in the car, which shocked me. I thought he would simply dismiss my claim completely. But, she reported, he was not being sexual with me that night in the blue Cadillac with Barbra singing Christmas carols. He was tickling me.

I wrote a letter to my parents. In part it read:

Most recently, I was devastated by the meeting of Kathy, me and Mom at your house. Not only was I hearing some things from Kathy for the first time which were difficult at best, but I was told that I was just like Dad, no different. And that my husband just wasn't taking care of me. I have heard that before, just as Kathy has. Thank God it isn't true. In all of my life, no one has ever cared about me completely the way Mark does and he has devoted a great deal of his adult life to helping me tiptoe through this minefield. How dare you say such a thing. I thank God every day for that man. He is the difference between me and some very bad things.

It is entirely clear to me that I will never get, from either of you, the "validation" I have been seeking for my own grief and pain over our family secret. It is the hurt child in me that wants that so badly from her mommy and daddy. But I am not a hurt child anymore and you are not acting like a mommy and daddy. I no longer give you the power to validate anything for me. And I will not waste one more ounce of energy trying so hard to show you my pain so that you can say it's okay.

I try not to feel shame but to feel proud of surviving the most serious breach of trust that a parent can perpetrate on their own child. Not being safe with your father is a terrible thing. Ask yourself, would you respond in the same way if it was someone other than the father, where it would be safer and not so complicated to feel the outrage? If it were a janitor, or a policeman, a babysitter or teacher? I am deeply ashamed of many of my feelings, feelings that Dad has ingrained in me and taught me by example. But I have learned it is not my fault. I am trying to do the work, and move through it.

So now I will never discuss the subject of sexual abuse in our family with either of you again. Please do not misconstrue my resolve to mean that I accept that you have done "everything you could." Because I do not accept that. In the most basic way, I cannot accept that Dad didn't know what he was doing was wrong and extremely damaging and it is very offensive to continually repeat that. It is also a very common defense among sexual offenders. It belittles the pain of the victims and takes all responsibility away from the offender. He ultimately claims "innocence." That's remarkable, don't you think, when it is our innocence that has been sacrificed?

CHAPTER TWENTY-FIVE

James told me about a friend of his who had recently purchased his family's business, urging me to consider taking charge of my own increasingly difficult work situation in the same manner. I listened carefully as he gently explained the possibilities, never telling me exactly what to do but just planting the seed. I began to believe that it was the only way out of the miserable combination of my complete responsibility for the daily operation of the business and the control it still gave my father over me, the access. I carefully planned how I would present it to my parents and set a meeting to discuss it. They had no inkling in advance of what was to come. Before I walked in the room, I called James for moral support, going over my strategy one more time.

We sat at the conference table in my office, me across from my two parents. I got right to the point. Not feeling like an employee, and not having any ownership stake offered to me thus far, I wished to buy the company right away. If that was not something they would consider, I would resign, no longer able to work under current conditions. My mother was horrified and immediately assumed that they could figure out some way to work this out that would leave them still in control. But my father looked at me with a twinkle in his eye as if to say, "You did it…you figured it out… you won." He was clearly proud of my long-term strategy and completely understood what had just happened. That pride was offset by the knowledge that he had lost. As I predicted, he was not willing to return to work and knew that without me, his company would have no value in a sale. He gave up. He agreed. On the spot. I also insisted that I be gifted one third of the company stock, which I had earned as a true partner from the very beginning, requiring me only to pay for two-thirds of the shares. He also agreed to that, acknowledging my contribution. At that very moment, symbolically, I had declared my independence. I knew it was why I had agreed to work with him in the first place. I was free.

I could have never predicted how this business and emotional achievement would play out in my life. But my mother gave me a clue. Still very angry at my demand to buy the business, literally robbing her of the ownership role she craved so much, she lashed out by telling me, once again and in a slightly different way, that I was "just like him."

CHAPTER TWENTY-SIX

The feelings, deeper now and more intense, had no place to go. They were rarely ever alone, stealing public moments here and there. He declared several times that he must stop seeing her as he was tired of being so miserable all the time. She did not agree but went along. It never lasted. While she was busy trying so hard to respect his decision, he changed his mind and called her office five times in one day to tell her. She finally took the last call. He told her if she hadn't, he was on his way over to see her. She saved the messages, locked them in the desk drawer, and kept them to remind her that he couldn't stay away from her. That he wanted her back. Had to have her back.

He began to insist on seeing her only if they could be totally alone, in private, to "visit" without worrying about who may see or hear them. She asked where that might take place and shuddered when he suggested a hotel room. That seemed impossible to her. But on two occasions, when she was missing him so much, she said she was ready to move forward with the relationship and offered to make the arrangements he required. He refused. Once he said they should just go back to their families and be grateful for all the good things in their lives. Although it hurt her, she was relieved and knew he was right. And, in her heart, she believed he was doing it for her. Putting her first, trying not to hurt her as deeply as he knew it would.

They met in the lobby of the same restaurant where she had met him that evening so long ago. He arrived and as they waited to be seated, he stood close behind her, his hands traveling down her back and onto her bottom, squeezing and rubbing, almost between her legs.

She moved closer, accepting him. Once seated, he asked her what was going on, forcing her to speak first as he always did. She asked if he thought they should be sleeping together. He said no, he didn't, but that didn't mean he didn't want to. She described her restlessness, which she knew he understood and had indulged so many times in his own life, and asked his advice. He became friend and counselor, doing just the right thing, describing how it usually isn't worth it and turns out to be no big deal, disappointing somehow. How it feels like it is really helping but in reality, it is only hurting. How he struggled every day of his life not to lead that life. How a young woman had recently suggested a liaison between them and he had turned her down, thinking of it as a sign of disrespect somehow. He said it could so easily ruin friendships and she said it was ruining theirs and they had not even had the "good stuff." He said she was wrong, that they were friends and that was the good stuff. She said she had been surprised to find out that she was really so much like him and he said he was beginning to see that, surprised also. She said that if she would decide to indulge those feelings, those powerful urges, that it would only be with him, it could never be with anyone else. He firmly and objectively said he probably would not even agree to that at this point. This was what she wanted and needed to hear, although her heart was breaking. He had to get back and left her. Just walked away. She was grateful somehow and working hard to accept his advice and move forward on her own, going back to her office and throwing herself into a very heavy work load.

An hour later he called. He wanted to come to her right away. He had to see her, even if just for a few moments, or all evening. She allowed his words and his desire to wash over her, sending her to the place she longed to be every moment. They agreed to meet the next morning but he called to say that he couldn't due to a schedule change. He seemed conflicted and depressed. She was crushed. He reconsidered and arranged to meet her at the park. She arrived first which was unusual, even suspicious. When he arrived, he wanted her to get in his car. She said, no, they should sit outside. He said for once they were going to be spontaneous, to get in the car. She did, knowing full well that something was happening. She was weakly resisting what she thought he had in mind. She was nervous and scared. So was he.

He drove them to a small motel very close by. He had stopped there on the way to the park to get them a room and already had the key. She loved that he had arranged this for her, what she had been unable to plan. She continued to resist, lovingly, not firmly, laughing nervously while he gently insisted. They walked up to Room 213. She couldn't believe she was doing it, only barely able to put one foot in front of the other. She was so afraid for herself, for them.

It was a small dark room with two beds, a TV and a bathroom. They each took a bed and sat, talking awkwardly. He said he had butterflies. Then he carefully explained what caused a golf ball to slice or how you could make it hook. He took off his tie and his shoes, pulled the bedspread off the pillows and laid back. She took off nothing. He pulled her legs over to him between the beds and began rubbing her legs, analyzing their quality and teaching her about the musculature. She was proud of her dancing legs and how much he seemed to enjoy and appreciate them. He spoke of massaging her, slowly and all over. She wanted that. But she couldn't let go. He spoke quietly, being ever so gentle with her. Finally he reached over to kiss her, softly at first and then with more need. Slowly he ran his hands over every part of her, concentrating completely. Then he pushed himself onto her, on her bed, as she spread her legs around his. He murmured about how much he had wanted to do that for so long. He looked into her eyes, stroking her face and her hair, continuing to kiss her on the mouth, the eyes, the neck and lower. His hands came around to her breasts and he rubbed them hard and firm. She responded completely, arching her back to be closer to him. He grabbed her back and pulled her even closer. He spoke to her quietly, calling her by name, suggesting they remove all their clothes. She said she looked better with her clothes on, still so nervous. He said he knew everyone did but they still should. He wanted to kiss her all over, slowly. He began to unbuckle her belt, asking if the t-shirt was a body suit. She said it was, with snaps. Wasn't that uncomfortable, he wanted to know? She said no. He unzipped her stretch jeans that clung to her hips and thighs like skin. He peeled them down, kissing each part as it was exposed. He didn't unsnap the body suit right away, instead reaching his hand inside of it and feeling her dampness, exploring. Then he unsnapped it and slowly pulled it up across her stomach, kissing her navel then following his kisses with his hands, continuing to pull it up, finally revealing her breasts. He had waited so long to see how one of them was covered by the birthmark which came down her arm and onto her hand. He looked long and hard at the two breasts, such a different color, and began to stroke and kiss the "strawberry" breast. He turned her over to follow it to her back, kissing every inch of the strawberry color to outline it with his lips as he had always promised he would do.

She now lay naked on her bed, with him still fully clothed. She took over, unbuttoning his shirt, pulling it off carefully, folding it on his bed. She pulled off his t-shirt, revealing the soft hair on his chest. She began to unhook his belt and unbutton and unzip his pants revealing the fullness of his sex. He was excited, hard and she kissed him there. As she pulled off his briefs and socks, she placed them on his bed with his shirt, leaving him fully naked. He was very at ease with his maleness. He wanted to share it with her, give it like a precious gift. She climbed onto him, straddling his pelvis and leaned forward to kiss him, feeling her breasts on his chest. His hands roamed all over her, stopping on her bottom, exploring to the front to find her opening. As he pushed two and then three fingers inside her, she sighed deeply. She lifted up so he could enter her. As he did so, he seemed to enlarge and grow inside of her, molding to her inner shape and filling her up perfectly. Gradually, she began to move on him in a gentle rhythm, then stretching out her legs on top of his, tightening her muscles so she could grab him inside of her and squeeze.

She then turned on her side so that he could mold to her body and enter her from behind, gently pushing and thrusting, kissing her shoulders and covering her breasts with his arms around her. She reached down to touch herself and his hand moved there to help. Her hips began to sway, responding to the gentle pressure between her legs, the fullness continuing until it began to sweep through her entire body. He grew and grew inside of her, talking to her, calling her by name, hands traveling all over her. She began to tense and shake, becoming vocal in her passion, finally releasing all feelings into a pounding, ecstatic orgasm. He smiled and held her tight, still hard and vital inside of her, giving her a chance to recover.

He then pulled her under him, thrusting into her vigorously. His tempo increased and he began to tighten his face as he drew closer to releasing. When he did, he exploded in her. They collapsed together, holding on, refusing to relinquish each other, sweaty and connected, joined. Finally.

She leaned against the bathroom door and watched intently as he buttoned his shirt and tied his tie in front of the mirror, putting himself back together perfectly. He then pressed her against the wall, running his hands through her hair, across her face and neck, studying her, looking hard into her eyes. At that moment, she belonged completely to him. He looked over at the tattered curtains, cheerfully declaring the place to be a dump. He said it was funny though, once you stepped inside, it became your palace.

That is what I wrote, in my usual third person narrative as though I were someone else, but not at all what happened. Everything starting with the part about "then he pushed himself onto her" was pure fantasy. I was so distressed at being unable to succumb to him that I went home and wrote the story as I imagined it would have happened if I had been able to go through with it. He was frustrated and dejected on that day, but never angry. Towards the painful end, he had sat on the bed and said that at least I now knew that this was not where I wanted to be or what I wanted to be doing. I asked him if it was where he wanted to be and what he wanted to be doing. He answered no. I did watch him put his tie back on and he did run his hands through my hair and over my face and neck. There was so much hurt and need on his face that I felt real pain. He took me back to the park to get my car and drove away immediately. I wondered if he was actually more hurt by all this than I was.

Despite the disaster in Room 213, I still felt that there would never be anyone else in my life that could fill that space that belonged only to him, the sexual space my father had created and nurtured in me and I had now given to James, his surrogate. They became one in what they taught me and expected me to learn about myself, how they viewed me as a sexual being, and what they wanted of me. Having sex with James would be the sex I hadn't had with my father. That is probably why I hadn't had it yet. This deeply troubling part of my life experience was probably as close as I would ever get to understanding how my father's life got so out of control. There was something so inherently wrong about it and I clung, by the smallest thread, to the notion that I was not my father's daughter. Just maybe, hopefully, I was not.

CHAPTER TWENTY-SEVEN

I delivered the written pages to James just to let him know that although I had not been able to go through with the planned activities in Room 213, I still played them out in my mind. I thought he deserved to know that. And honestly, I knew that it would keep him in the game. That evening, I was incredibly restless and left the house with the Walkman feeding carefully selected music into my head, chosen to reflect my state of mind. I put the studio keys in my pocket on the off chance that classes might be over for the evening, allowing me to go in for a while. It was dark when I arrived, the parking lot softly lit by decorative lamps. Sometimes I was afraid there at night, but not this time. I sat on the curb with Crosby, Stills and Nash singing "Lady of the Island" straight into my ears. "Holding you close undisturbed before the fire, the pressure in my chest when you breathe in my ear, we both knew this would happen when you first appeared." I was intoxicated by this song just as I was in 1969 when I first heard it. I went into the studio. With shadows from outside light coming in, the room was alive with movement. I couldn't bring myself to turn on the lights, wanting only to exist in this moving room, wanting to move freely myself with no particular purpose.

Up until recently, the dance studio had meant something different to me. There were students to teach, classes to take, dances to choreograph, rehearsals to run. All work. Now I entered only for myself, grateful for every single moment of training I had ever endured. My body looked different in my old leotards, fuller, but I still had the thin, long look of a dancer and a strong sense of my body. It was the first time I had felt free enough to wear a leotard without a bra and didn't even mind if the lower scoop necks revealed my strawberry birthmark. This was a part of myself that I could now accept, even embrace. I loved the feeling of my body against the thin, clingy material, knowing I could simply pull the leotard down over my shoulders to expose my breasts. I sometimes placed a chair in the corner of the room and imagined that James was sitting there, watching me dance. He would come to me and pull the leotard off my shoulders, not minding my sweat, stroking and kissing my body with music still playing, all a part of the dance. I would respond completely, kissing him and pulling my tights down from my hips so he could touch me everywhere. He would enter me in this dream of a dance, my clothes heaped on the wooden floor, but he would remain fully clothed, needing to have me immediately. Tonight I moved his chair to the center of the room and let "Lady of the Island" play.

The music took me back to my college campus in 1969. I was only 16 years old and taught classes in the school's dance curriculum. I had a key to the beautiful studio on the old, conservative Alabama campus. Because I was so young and felt out of place, I often spent weekend evenings on that wood floor listening to that piece of music, dancing. Those feelings came flooding back to me as I sat on the chair in the middle of the dark studio. I was just as carried away by the emotion then as now. But things were so much simpler then. I had never been with a man. The idea of being held close undisturbed before the fire was a romantic image with no understanding of the complications of having had sex before being held. No understanding of the difficulty of trying to decide when sex should happen at all. When was the man appropriately honorable yet swept away by desire for you? Would he stay with you? Was he using you? Was it really true that men just took sex from women thereby suggesting that women were always giving something away, giving something up? If you gave it away, could you ever get it back? What about performance, orgasms, one or more, or none? What about pregnancy? Should you even have sex if it might produce a child with someone you wouldn't want to raise a child with? In those days, I just danced and expressed myself and dreamed about what someday might be.

It was obviously recital time as I could see the flecks of glitter on the floor and plastic bags with costume pieces stored in the corner. There were stick-on stars for good behavior and certificates for student of the month. There were tiny pink ballet slippers carelessly left behind by four-year-olds after class which had that distinctive smell of Capezio leather. There were silver barrettes and rubber bands that had fallen out of baby fine hair in the frenzy of turns across the floor and visions of swans and fairies. There were pictures on the walls of beautiful ballerinas on toe shoes with perfect turnout and strong, high arches in their feet. In all these images was the not yet mature girl who was still free to allow her inner life to live and grow. This while the boys were out roughhousing, getting dirty, scraped and bumped. What happens when the two finally collide, perhaps in a car on a weekend night? Is that where her inner life begins to fade? Or perhaps it's when it is her father in the car with her instead. Does she begin to lose her choices? Does she begin to lose herself?

I responded by becoming strong and always in control, never risking a serious mistake that I might regret, building careful and intelligent walls around my inner core to instinctively protect and preserve its beauty. And I excelled, making sure that everyone always admired my achievements. I would always do the right thing and do it perfectly. I would mold my own life and feelings to that goal. I would not have sex until I met the man I could completely trust with my core and knew it may not ever happen at all.

When I found my lifetime partner, he met every qualification. I knew I could trust him and I was right. I never felt like I was giving anything up, but instead I was learning and growing and stretching to allow him access to me. He inspired that, a beautiful mentor.

But I was beginning to feel that I had missed something, going from the wildly dangerous world of my father to the safe, secure ultimately mature world of Mark. I was starting to unravel the sexual feelings that had always been so unsafe and inappropriate, carefully hidden for so long. Mark associated those emerging feelings with an unhealthy connection to my upbringing and did not encourage them, opting to keep us on a healthy, married version of sex, love and the responsibility of family life. He was becoming increasingly threatened by my awakening, often feeling overwhelmed and trapped. And yet the feelings continued to come over me like a tidal wave, an image that inhabited my dreams. He treated me like this was an inconvenient period I was going through from which I would one day hopefully recover. But I did not want to miss a moment of it. James wanted to assist with my awakening and was a completely different kind of mentor. But the profound sense of loyalty and commitment I felt to Mark and my family and the rightness of our lives prevented me from fully exploring these powerful feelings. I had taken it very far, but could not connect to the actual sex part, which felt like the ultimate betrayal and the one thing that would ally me with my father as his daughter forever. I knew that step would change everything. I was afraid of losing control, of losing everything, of not losing control. And I wondered how I would know if the risk must be taken. What if I chose wrong, either way?

CHAPTER TWENTY-EIGHT

I opened my eyes before him, as I did most every morning, instantly awake, planning what I would get up and get to. But this particular morning, Mother's Day, I alternated between closing my eyes and watching Mark sleep. I was fascinated by the twitching of his face, the emotion that seemed to come and go across it, and the way his penis was so active, sometimes standing straight up under the sheet. I wondered what was going on inside of him, just as I often did when he was awake. He was so beautiful to look at. The day before had been our wedding anniversary, eighteen years married and four more living together. I was nineteen when I fell madly in love with him at first sight. I completely trusted him, he had never hurt me, and I knew he never would. It was as it should be, if you could ever accept it.

Our two sons were sleeping right across the hall. I loved that feeling, knowing we were all safe in our home. I was not the least bit unhappy in my life with these three. I loved them all completely.

On the evening of our anniversary, we went to our favorite restaurant where we were known, welcomed and treated well. It was very familiar in its routine, just as we were, and we loved those evenings out together. I always dressed in a way that made me feel very sexy and sensual, often skipping the underwear and letting my long hair go wild. Sometimes we would end up at my office where, without ever turning the lights on, he would make love to me on my big desk, in my executive chair, on the conference table, or even the floor. Sometimes he didn't feel like it, though I always did. I loved those times; they were the best of everything with excitement, physical intimacy, yet the trust and familiarity.

I had planned a surprise for him and dressed for it in advance. I wore an off the shoulder red leotard with no bra. I covered that with my favorite thin flannel shirt which slid off one shoulder. Then my stretch jeans, which moved almost like tights. After dinner, I took him to the dance studio. It was easy since I always drove home because he drank and I didn't. I placed him in a chair and danced two pieces for him in the same clothes in which I had dined with him. He was very moved by this gesture, hugging me afterwards and letting his hands roam over me. I always wanted that to lead to more but tonight it was okay.

When we got home and in bed, I lay next to him wearing only his old tattered t-shirt, big as a dress, which made me feel wonderful. We watched TV and he rubbed my bare bottom, which I loved, for a long, long time. He was a little too drunk, full and tired to have sex, so I touched myself with my own hand, he covered it with his and helped me come, rubbing my breast and talking quietly to me in one ear. We fell asleep together, really together. It was one of the best times we had ever had coping with the problem of me wanting and needing sexual attention and him unable or unwilling to give it. We were both content. I thought of this the next morning watching him sleep and was overwhelmed with love for him. I finally got up anyway, wanting to stay but not wanting to create a possibly difficult sexual demand when he awoke.

It was Mother's Day and my three Dutch boys made me feel very special, treating me to cards, gifts and hugs. We visited my parents briefly and I found a box of old photographs taken when I was very young, many that I had never seen before. I was fascinated by my own demeanor in the images. I saw a natural radiance, a luminous look that I felt I was beginning to rediscover, an essence that had been lost for such a long time.

When we came home, I danced at the studio for an hour or so. It was the first time that I had not been grieving in my dancing, working something out, calming anxieties, or expressing pain and longing. Instead I danced with joy in my heart, free for the moment. Happy. I wore no make-up and I felt beautiful. I felt loved.

Suddenly I was so glad that I had not taken my clothes off in Room 213. So damned glad.

CHAPTER TWENTY-NINE

Iknew I had taken a huge step by allowing James to read my account of what didn't happen in Room 213. I knew it would gradually work on him. We hadn't spoken in a week and I was proud of each day that I didn't indulge my urge to call him. Like an alcoholic who can mark one more day of sobriety on the calendar. I knew it was an addiction, my need for him. When my life had been so tight and under control, I had no addictions. It was hard to get used to and made me feel very human, helped me understand human weakness. James called it the need to step off my pedestal and join everyone else. I could not imagine being well enough to make it without him for a month, or a year, or even a day actually, probably because I had not yet admitted the need to. It had been fascinating to realize how worked up I must have been in order to get myself into a position to even go to Room 213, how much it meant to me, and the extended frustration of indulging those feelings without consummating them with him. But when I returned from that room and wrote down what didn't happen, but in my mind should have, it almost had the effect of having gone through with it. Now I pretty much only thought of getting back there to take a nap with him, to be close, not to have sex. I felt like we already had. I was quite sure he did not.

I felt my cheeks go hot when he called before I succumbed to making the call myself. Normally that would thrill me knowing how much he would prefer to have waited for my call but couldn't quite be patient enough. It would have been a small but satisfying victory proving I was winning the battle for control between us. The upper hand in the psychological game. But I knew it meant he couldn't wait, that my story was working on him, and he wanted to see me, touch me and make my fantasy his reality. I wondered why that filled me with so much dread rather than the usual excitement. He wanted me to come to his office, describing in detail where I would stand, what I would be wearing and not wearing, how he would touch my bare legs, and move up to satisfy me. I didn't know why this fantasy of his was so different than my own fantasy about which I had written in detail just one week ago. His voice continued to weave the details of my hoped for visit and I realized that this was a serious game and he was a very advanced player. I made an excuse and promised to get back to him but as soon as I hung up, I knew that I would not make that trip to his office. Not after the relief my writing had given me and the wonderful, peaceful day I had just had with my family. No, I would definitely not go.

My father had taught me, by example, how to use every ounce of my intelligence to control, manipulate, and prevail in every situation. I had learned my lesson so well that I eventually became better at it than him, ultimately gaining the very control that had once been his evil weapon against all of us. I was struck by the similarities between James and my father, both powerful and controlling, leading a secret life with other women while married and totally believing that they had the right somehow. My father had once told me how he did not think that he had hurt his family by having his secret life because he was still a good husband, good provider, and good father. That he simply had the need and the capacity to have more. The only mistake he had made was finally admitting his indiscretions. He regretted that now, he had said. I was totally disgusted by his selfish ravings at the time, hating him for deciding what did and didn't hurt our family, what did and didn't destroy our mother, what did and didn't cause him to treat my sister like a mistress.

And here I was now, involved with a man just like him in so many ways. Myself being one of the other women in his life, being the potential cause of so much hurt and shame. What drove me to this place? Maybe I was transferring my rage from my father to him, teasing him, luring him, but never letting him have me, just to prove to him that this one time in his life, he couldn't have his way with a woman. But how did I become so caught up in it? I had denied my sexuality for so long because my father's obsession with it disgusted me so. But when I broke free of him, my natural instincts came forward and I thought them to be clean and strong and healthy. When my husband pulled away, I responded intensely to the sexual attention paid to me by James. I thought it my right somehow after such a long period of denial of these feelings, but then didn't my father think it was his right also? I had strong moments of believing that I was really just like him anyway and became determined to prove it. Those times made me feel so worthless. And yet I could not turn away.

But sitting in my big executive chair with the phone to my ear, listening to him feel so comfortable and entitled to describing his fantasy to me, knowing it was okay with me, put me in a spin. I was confused. After hanging up, I left right away. As I opened my office door, which I had closed for privacy, all of my employees had left and I was alone. I felt stupid and isolated, inhuman somehow. How much better it would have been to have said good night to everyone, close up shop, and go home to my family.

When I did get home, I was completely insensitive to how

tired Mark looked and instead wanted him to make love to me. He didn't, even after I sent him the usual strong signals. I became restless and began to subtly provoke him, punish him, sending the clear message that he was not satisfying me. How damaging a pattern this had become for us and how clearly I suddenly saw it.

I wandered over to the studio, did not have the energy to dance legitimately, instead sang in the dark, feeling strange and insecure. I leaned myself against a cool, concrete wall and brought myself to a strong orgasm, feeling my way through his office fantasy in my mind, allowing it to happen to me inside. Even though I loathed myself at that moment, I still vowed to call him first thing the next morning and tell him my version of his office fantasy. When I returned home, my husband expressed concern over my safety being out alone that late at night. I was cool and unappreciative to his genuine caring.

After falling asleep for a few hours, I awoke in a cold sweat, reliving the phone conversation, my stomach filling with acid. I was horrified that I had contemplated reproducing his behavior the next day. My feeling of contamination illuminated my shame. I wondered if it would be enough this time. Enough for me to stop.

I cried, trying to withhold my sobs so that I would not awaken Mark sleeping next to me. He did wake up and offered to listen if I wanted to talk, not insisting, of course. I said no, I couldn't. He cuddled up to me, rubbed my back, and asked what he could do for me. This was so unlike him, this affectionate support and physical comfort. Although it had an immediate soothing effect on me, it also made me feel so sad and guilty. Thinking that somehow I could cleanse myself of all the shame and misery, I got up and took a long, hot shower, covering every inch of my body with the scent I had worn since I was a teenager. I returned to bed where he welcomed me warmly and held me until I fell asleep, once asking if his closeness was bothering me.

I had suddenly seen the amazing clarity of Mark's love for me. How unselfish it really was. How he knew so much about what I was going through, how he knew I had to do it, how he hoped that I would figure it out before I destroyed myself. And us. Again, I was overwhelmed with love for him. I knew what I had to do. I didn't know if I could.

CHAPTER THIRTY

Badly shaken, I made no phone calls to James the following day, unable to bear the emotion of it. The long busy work day was a relief and a welcome distraction.

He called the next day, firmly telling me that he had cleared his calendar for Friday afternoon and felt that I should do the same. I said I would let him know. His last comment was that Friday was open and it was going to stay that way. I knew it was hard for him to be so assertive and risk yet one more refusal from me. But Mark and I had a long standing date to go to the movies whenever I could get away from the office on Friday afternoons. And it would be impossible to explain my lack of availability for that outing without creating a larger than life lie, which I was unwilling to do.

On Thursday afternoon, James called to see if Friday was going to happen. I said it didn't look good. But he wanted me to say yes so bad. It wasn't the usual proposition filled with playful mischief, instead a real requirement to see me, be with me. I understood that because I often felt exactly the same way. I promised to still try to arrange it.

Later that evening, I was overcome with the need to see him, go to him. It was close to one of those few times I had experienced before where I wildly and ridiculously thought I might call him at home. I knew that calling him at home was completely out of control, and I didn't really think I would do it. But how easy it seemed it would be. What if he did answer and they could quickly agree to meet somewhere right away, right then, and their powerful and overwhelming desire could be satisfied. It seemed more important than anything else, and justifications for such behavior were plentiful and totally manufactured.

He called twice on Friday morning but I had to say it just wasn't going to happen. Having to refuse him was so painful and felt so wrong that I was traumatized while driving to meet Mark at the theatre. How could I possibly feel guilty for lying to James so I could meet my husband? It turned out we had the time wrong for the movie anyway and had to abandon the whole outing. This sent me into an emotional tailspin, thinking that if I had just told the large lie, I would be with James right then.

The rest of the day was a miserable blur. My confusion and conflict was so deep and pervasive that I was barely able to function. I left James a voice mail message saying I was leaving work at 520, thoroughly exhausted, and was sorry that we weren't able to get together. I wasn't sure how long I could continue to go on this way.

CHAPTER THIRTY-ONE

Mark continued to take care of me, support me and treat me more affectionately than ever before. But he was becoming more and more withdrawn from sex. In fact, I felt that he was showing me more affection as some sort of trade off for not wanting to have sex. I did not seem able to affect him at all and we were limited to having sex only when his natural cycle of desire resurfaced. And that seemed to be less and less often. He teased me about being ready and moist at all times, even with no preparation, and I loved to let him use me for a quick sexual encounter but regretted that it did not allow me to have my own orgasm with him, to share that with him. And I knew it would be quite a while before I got another chance. I had been taking care of myself with increasing regularity. I used to be careful about when I would do that, trying to predict when he would want to have sex so that I could save a nice orgasm for him. But lately it didn't seem to matter much. I mostly thought of James when I made myself come, knowing how much he wanted to share that with me, share everything with me. How much he wanted me. I felt that being desired in that way was one of the most important parts of myself. An absolute requirement.

Saturday morning, Mark got up first, slipping out of bed, getting dressed, to let me know that there would be no sex once again. The feeling I had when I watched him dress and walk out of our room was so devastating to me that it seemed unbearable. Our pattern in the past year was exactly the same. He avoided our sexual encounters completely and I would work very hard at accepting and understanding that, trying not to put pressure on him, relying on my own hand and my strong, sensual and passionate inner life. But after a certain period of time, maybe ten days or so, something clicked inside of me and I had to talk to him about it.

On this morning I tried to be gentle and non-judgmental. I suggested that my impression was that he was feeling totally non-sexual again and he admitted that was true. I thought maybe he could go to the doctor to eliminate a physiological cause for the problem. He became irritated and upset like he did every time. I cried. We weren't compatible in this way, he said. But we agreed that we had virtually no other problems. We talked about living apart for a while but I saw that as a time when I would experiment and find out the real priority of this in my life. He said he would not be so anxious to take me back if that was what I would do. I would stand by him indefinitely in this way if he was willing to admit this was a problem and seek solutions. But he refused to see a therapist and admitted that he did not wish to tell a doctor that he did not have enough interest in sex to satisfy me. I understood that but felt that the seriousness of this problem between us should take precedence over the temporary discomfort of embarrassment with a physician. This time was different in some ways than the countless others because he really was slipping away, and accepting it. He simply didn't have much sex drive, he said, and that was okay with him. He hoped that I would get over this exaggerated need of mine. I told him that I did not wish to get over it, that I had worked hard to get in touch with that part of myself and would not simply wish it away. Instead I wished to explore it and enjoy it and bask in it. That made him feel threatened and impotent.

Oh, the irony of it. I had felt too unsafe throughout my life to express that part of myself as a result of my father's inappropriate sexual influence. As a woman, I had fought my way to emotional freedom, and as a result, my body and sensual spirit awakened with a vengeance. And yet that process took away the desire for me of the only man I had, the only man I loved. He thought it another unfortunate symptom of my sexually abusive past. I didn't. His stoic stability did have its advantages, but I did not see how I could continue to live with so little sexual expression available to me. It made me constantly miserable.

It didn't help that James was so sensual and emotional and desired me more than anything. His gentle pressure worked on me and certainly did not help my situation at home. I longed to let him come to me, to give in to those feelings, to find out what it was all about. My biggest fear was the he would give up on me before I could find my way to him and would not want me anymore. I knew that could happen at any time.

Mark and I didn't go out for our usual Saturday night dinner after the miserable morning discussion about his lack of interest in sex with me. Instead our early evening frustration turned into a long talk about the problem. Somehow it wandered to my interest in exploring my sexual feelings with another man. He let me know that he could not accept that, even in the context of a separation and if I chose that, I would be closing the door on our life together. In my frame of mind, that meant that he would not ever help me discover that part of myself, and no one else was allowed to either. I was angry and resentful, feeling sorry for how trapped I felt. I promised him that I was not yet sleeping with anyone else and also that if I decided I must, I would leave first so that he would not be in a position of being deceived or "cuckolded" as he was fond of calling it.

I didn't tell him how close I was coming each and every day, that I had been to Room 213, how intimately I allowed James to speak to me and think of me, how I had shared my written pages with him holding nothing back, how valiantly I fought every day to avoid finally letting it all go. What a terrible price I was paying for all of that.

He still allowed me to come close in bed that night where I fell asleep. As long ago as I could remember, no matter what was going on between us, he never turned me away emotionally, never judged me, never made me feel bad about myself. I was only now beginning to realize how valuable that was to me. And how much I was going to need that in the future.

As we awoke, in the dim light of the early morning, he moved over to hold me close. I said I had thought about it and there was only one answer to our problem for now. We had to go through a period of celibacy. For one month to start with. That way I would always know that there was no chance we would be having sex and he would feel no pressure. He didn't take me seriously but instead I could feel him getting aroused. He agreed to the plan, but starting tomorrow. Once he began to make love to me, I had no power to refuse although I knew this was a time I should. I could never remember saying no to him. Never. For the first time in recent memory, I did not feel like I could go with the sex. It did not carry me away as it usually did. At one point I could only think about what it would be like if it was James, wishing it was, wishing I had the courage to make it so.

I got up and dressed in my dance clothes to go to the studio to try to process all my bad feelings. I put on a bare leotard with wool tights rolled at the waist, held with a belt. Suddenly and unexpectedly, we began to discuss things like never before with a sense of honesty that was disarming and frightening, transcending our behaviors and moving to the bare and terrifying truth. It all began to spill out of me, how I had seen a film the afternoon before and even though it had been about an alcoholic woman and her relationship with her husband, I felt it was really about me. I, too, was an addict. I had become addicted to sex, to sexual feelings, and to satisfying them and it was controlling at least my inner life and certainly beginning to affect my daily life and relationships as well. After all, I had been raised by a sexually addicted man who taught by example that you could take what you need, and then you could control and manipulate the potential damage to others. Maybe I was just like him. I was so close to living the exact same life as my father. The woman in the film had impressed upon her husband that even though she lived in a nice house, had two beautiful children, a loving husband, and a successful career, she also had the potential to be the woman in her support group who had been living on the park bench with a bottle for the past three years. And for the first time, my husband heard from me that I was just one fuck away from stepping over the line and living the life of my father, hanging on by my fingernails each and every day to avoid that. He asked wasn't it like children of alcoholics who swore they would never drink because of the damage done by alcoholic parents? And then never did? Couldn't I just do it that way and promise it would never happen to me? I explained that I could never be satisfied not knowing if I could really walk away from it to be free from it forever because I had never allowed myself to go there and the struggle to prevent it was about to knock me out completely. Perhaps if I just went there, I would find out that my fear was unfounded and I didn't want it, didn't need it, and could come back to the other side to finally find peace. But what if I found that I could live on the other side and wanted to? Then I would declare my addiction and treat it as such. But doing so, going there to find out, could be a risk to my marriage from which we might never recover.

I stood up, practically hysterical by this time, in tears, and pointed to myself in the mirror. In the glass was my dance trained body in leotard and tights, and I screamed that sex was what my body was about to me now. For all those years, I hid myself in high necklines and flannel pajamas, never allowing myself to be seen as a sexual being. Now I had shot over to the other extreme, seeing my body as only that, after I had supposedly freed myself from the powerful control of my father's disturbed perspective. I wanted my body to be more than that, more than a sexual instrument. But I didn't know how to make it so. I could see by his pained expression that he knew exactly what I was saying, not that he could relate, but he could understand. I spoke of how I got up every morning and made the right choices but how hard I had to fight to do so. And he didn't even know about the pressure I had from James. Always pulling me to the other side. And I couldn't tell him. I said I wasn't even sure I could possibly go for a month without sex, how afraid I was of a month without sex. Like wanting a drink, needing a drink. A fix. I knew that James understood because he was my partner in this addiction, or at least wanted to be. In a way, there was comfort in that for me, knowing that I could have sex with a person who was as obsessed with it as I was. Two of a sorry kind. Lately I had been feeling so ashamed of Mark's awareness of my devastating need, totally overshadowing his own need, and obviously causing his complete sexual withdrawal from me. The damage done.

As painful as it all was, I felt better. I had never actually said any of that out loud, or consciously realized it. I only knew for sure that right now the intensity of the conflict that I perceived as right vs. wrong, healthy vs. unhealthy, self-control vs. indulgence was controlling my existence. I knew that I could probably avoid calling James from my office the next day but also knew he would eventually call me. And that I would float with him to that place where all I could think about would be our desire and how it would be satisfied if only I could allow it.

CHAPTER THIRTY-TWO

I awoke early in the morning, the first day of a month without sex according to the celibacy agreement. I was restless and terrified. It would never work. Mark stirred as I tossed and turned. He reached over to try to settle me but his touch only made things worse. He became very interested, hard and responsive. He seemed surprised and pleased with himself and assumed that I would, as usual, override our brand new agreement and give in to him. Assumed I was that weak on the very first day. But I was tired of being controlled by my desire, even more tired of that than not having my own desire satisfied. I kissed him, enjoyed his roving hands, and teased him. Then I arose from bed to start the day. He made some remark about how it wouldn't be so bad to just go ahead and do it, trying to disguise his real need to now that I wasn't available, making it sound like it was really for me. I gently refused, saying that I was like this every morning, all the time, and if we went back to the old way, nothing would ever change. Just no, not this time. I had never said no before. He fell back asleep and I got in the shower and had a big orgasm all by myself.

Sure enough, James called by midday wanting to know when we could meet. I put him off with talk of my workload but we both knew it was a smokescreen. Having, over the weekend, discovered that I was addicted to him and our sexual connection, I thought it best after having resisted my husband for the first time that morning to just say no to everything that day. For myself. He was frustrated and hurt but I stayed strong. And remote.

When I saw Mark again later that day, he was still excited and again kissed me, caressed me and showed me how excited he was. I smiled, responded, but declined to lift my skirt for him. How enjoyable for me to be the one who was wanted.

The effect of my new determination to control this powerful thing rather than let it control me was a wonderful relief, making me realize for the first time how truly victimized I had been by my desire for such a long time. It felt great but I assumed it was probably temporary.

And it was. The very next day James cleared his calendar for me, stating sarcastically that whatever time he suggested would most likely not work out for me anyway. But I went. I drove right over. I wanted to share my obsessive state of mind with him, my feelings, how they were driving me mad, and how out of control I felt. And to assure him that it wasn't that I didn't want to be with him, instead it was quite the opposite. How could I ever manage the real thing when I couldn't even handle such limited contact?

I tried to concentrate while giving my little speech although he was so delighted that I was there that he didn't really seem to care what I had to say. When I said how preoccupied I was, he suggested simply that I take it in stages and work each step out along the way. I apologized for the obvious discomfort and frustration I was causing. He said it was kind of exciting to continue right to the edge and then pull back. But what about how it could make a person feel so crazy and unbalanced? Or blind, he added, smiling. I knew what he meant. It was the same for me.

His lighthearted indulgence of my need to talk about things again and again, rather than do things, was such a relief that I felt wonderful when I left. Most likely it was more to do with how I allowed him to put his hand under my skirt and explore between my legs, skillfully and with extreme concentration and enjoyment.

CHAPTER THIRTY-THREE

I believed that this reckless behavior was not just a woman straying from her husband and family, but necessary emotional investigation, which could not be skipped. I knew that Mark could forgive me for delving into such dangerous territory to find out something so essential about myself. In fact, I was pretty sure he already knew somehow. I did not believe that he would forgive me if I actually slept with another man which was a different thing altogether. That fine line meant everything to me. And I guarded it at all costs.

James called asking if I could spend some time with him in the afternoon. I made it clear that whatever he had in mind, I was not agreeing to anything in particular. He said that napping and visiting were enough. When I expressed doubt as to the truthfulness of that statement, he admitted a severe case of performance anxiety that he would work out slowly. He told me to make the arrangements this time and leave a message telling him where we would meet. I begged him not to ask me to do that but he insisted, telling me to think of it as an adventure. I foolishly agreed.

Somehow I forced myself to drive back to the same dump as before, remembering that he had taught me to pay cash and never use my real name. In a sad but hopeful sign, I registered using Patti, my childhood name, and Michael's last name, giving my high school address in Virginia. Attaching Michael's name to this insane action somehow gave it a feeling of emotional safety. Doing so made me feel innocent and protected, if only for a brief moment. James didn't mention that they would ask me for identification after I had made up the name. So I had to lie about having recently moved to the Valley and married, thus my new last name. I bore up to the clerk's suspicious look, took the room key, and moved my car to a parking space in front of Room 204.

Arriving first, with lunch in hand, to the room I had chosen and paid for empowered me to be in charge of what would happen in it. As instructed, I left a voice mail for James saying where he could find me. The room was smaller and brighter than the last, but with only one bed this time. I ate my lunch by the window but didn't open the drapes. I lay on the bed and watched a soap opera, almost falling asleep, feeling strangely relaxed and content. It made me wonder if I wouldn't have been better off just enjoying the room myself without the inevitable stress of what was about to happen.

Even so, I was relieved to see him when he arrived, looking handsome and happy, but charmingly nervous. I returned to my already established place curled up on the bed. He sat down next to me and rubbed my feet and legs. This was his way of staking out what I was wearing, trying to determine what he had to contend with if he got lucky. I had chosen pants on this day, not wanting to make it so easy for him to slip his hand under one of my short skirts. Underneath I wore a one piece lace body suit that I knew he would love.

He wanted us to take off some of our clothes, but I declined. He lay with me for a few minutes, curling up close, stroking my long loose hair, and kissing me thoroughly. He asked my permission to remove his trousers. I didn't answer, suddenly confused and uncertain. He got up anyway, removed his pants and carefully folded them over the chair. But he left his shirt on which mostly covered his briefs. I knew he didn't want to but it was his concession to my reluctance.

He told me to turn over so he could rub my back which I found very appealing until I realized it was only going to be quick and superficial, as he was obviously displeased to be feeling the fabric of my clothes rather than my bare skin. But I was still determined to allow this experience to teach me about myself and my feelings and it was too soon to stop, even though it was tempting to jump up and get the hell out of there.

He lay on top of me, mimicking what we would be doing if we were nude and having sex. He had always told me we would go slow and on this very day had repeated that nothing had to happen. But I had been right. Very early on he announced that his performance anxiety was taking care of itself and I knew what that meant. My attempts to go back to the visiting and napping scenario completely failed. His need continued to press me. At one point it almost turned into a physical struggle and I worried that he might not release me. I made two trips to the bathroom for relief and to look at my face in the mirror. I forced myself to continue. I had to know.

I began to realize that many of the things that felt natural to me from years of intimate behavior with my husband were so much more pleasurable within our long-term relationship than in this secret, stressful environment, designed only to create an opportunity for sex. And how very performance oriented it was. We had long since given up chatting about families, jobs, daily struggles. It had all come to be about this moment. Having access to each other's bodies, using penises, vaginas, breasts, tongues and all the tools of sexual encounters. Suddenly I wondered if I had all that and a hundred times more with my husband, why would

I need to duplicate such a narrow part of that life with someone else? And at such great risk? It seemed redundant, and unlike what I expected, there was nothing magical about the way he touched me.

I had commented when he first arrived that several men had watched me park my Volvo wagon, which he called my "wifemobile," and that I assumed it must be an oddity for them to see such a nice car and a woman dressed as I was in such a place. He said no, that was exactly the kind of car they were used to seeing, suggesting that it was well-to-do housewives who were spending time in places like this, doing exactly what we were doing, only more. I was not in that category, I thought. I had a spectacular husband, a very successful life, and an unfortunate problem that led me to this place today. And I was relieved and overjoyed to discover that the long awaited, isolated sexual experience was giving me so little pleasure. In fact, I was barely able to tolerate it when he began to insist that I move my hand to his legs, between his legs. I knew he was suggesting that we take care of each other without intercourse. And when I was on top of him, stretched out over his body, moving in rhythm, I was upset to discover that my body was responding and preparing to climax. I immediately pulled back to avoid and resist that, knowing if I came for him, I would feel I had given that very intimate part of myself that I now absolutely did not want to give.

I forced myself to feel the feelings totally and completely so that I would never forget that I had made myself completely available for the choice that had consumed me for so long. I watched him as he moved from position to position, partially participating to keep it going but knowing that I wasn't really a part of all this. When he said that he wanted to feel my skin, my body, virtually begging me to remove my clothing and get into bed with him, I had no desire for that to happen. None whatsoever. And I felt myself emerge and take over, knowing for sure that I was not my father, feeling ashamed that I had to plummet to this moment to find out. But I knew that my husband would forgive me, that God would forgive me, and that I would forgive myself. And I would be rewarded for caring enough about myself to put an end to this intolerable pain and suffering.

Despite my repeated refusal to remove my clothing, James deftly began to unbuckle my belt and unzip my pants. I allowed him to move his hands up and down my lace bodysuit, giving him access to my bare skin, breasts and pelvis. At one point, he lifted my blouse up enough to kiss my right breast, the strawberry one that fascinated him so. His hands wandered down between my legs. Just as he was about to slip his fingers inside of me, I pulled away, vowing to myself that no one besides my husband was going to have access to inside of me.

I slid off to the bathroom and put myself back together. Returning to sit on the edge of the bed, I brushed my hair and prepared to leave. He pulled me back once more and again I responded, letting him run his hands over my entire body. This I did for myself, sealing all of the feelings inside of me. Making sure. He moved his hand to his crotch, saying he was going to stay and finish by himself. I said I knew he would. He asked if I would like to help him get started. I said no, I was started up enough for the both of us and had to go. I told him I loved him, which I did.

I knew at that moment that he had been my road to self-realization, gently bringing me to this moment, showing me patience and respect along the way, already knowing in his own way what I needed to find out about myself. I felt bad for hurting him the way I knew I had but I also knew how many women he had hurt and used in his own life. Maybe I was his penance.

So I got into my turbo wifemobile, drove myself away and wondered how I could ever face my husband without dying of the pain of it. I wanted to call him right away but resisted, feeling it was disrespectful to him at that moment. I returned to my office and was amazed to discover that nothing had really changed and no one seemed to know about my afternoon. I'm certain I looked pale and exhausted, which I was. Completely emotionally exhausted. I found it a great relief to talk about business and solve problems with co-workers. It felt strong and good and right and worthy.

When I returned home, Mark seemed to be surrounded by a soft, yellow aura. I wanted to step right into that light and bask in it forever, hoping I still had the right. He asked about my day and I said it was fascinating and that, someday, I would tell him about it. Perhaps in a year or so. In his usual way, he did not demand or press, but looked deep inside me, knowing.

I had a short, intense workout, sweating out the earlier experience and couldn't wait to shower. I lingered, washing and rewashing every part of my body that had been subjected to Room 204. I brushed my teeth, hoping that fatal diseases were not transmitted through kissing.

CHAPTER THIRTY-FOUR

When I awoke next to Mark the following morning, we talked about the usual things. Spontaneously we began to respond to each other and I was overwhelmed by a strong urge to love him completely and with fierce passion, in the way that I had not been able to love in Room 204. But there was the celibacy agreement. Mark suggested a temporary truce, but I wouldn't. Instead we indulged in the activities that were allowed without breaking the agreement and it felt exciting and new.

Later I tried to call James. Not because I needed him but because I was truly worried about him, about what I had put him through. He didn't answer all day. I hoped he was okay and could only imagine how difficult it had been for him, as emotional as he was. During that interlude in Room 204, I actually felt sorry for him. I had been drawn to him because I knew that he understood my constant craving, only he would most likely never be free of it as I someday hoped to be. He had once revealed to me that as a boy, he had been sexually abused by a neighbor woman. I believed that this woman had taught him to please her and he had learned his lessons well. I also imagined it was a skill that served him well on his own road to success.

I knew that he would most likely never conquer that part of himself that I refused to allow to continue to grow and fester inside of me like a tumor. I felt that something inside of me had died in the motel room that day, that I had hunted it down and killed it. I knew in some ways I would miss it. How I wished he did not have to live with it anymore either because I was sure that his repeated interludes to attempt to satisfy the insatiable need were sad and depressing. And I was also sure that my final refusal in Room 204 simply illuminated his pain. He knew that I would walk away better and stronger, and that he would be left behind.

CHAPTER THIRTY-FIVE

But there was still the raw emotion. The part of me that simply could not fit into the intellectual exercise or the psychological awareness that I committed myself to so completely after the certainty of my response to Room 204. Despite my best intentions, the game continued where it left off, like a movie that went on way too long, making you want nothing more than to head for the exit but unable to go until you saw how it all turned out.

Prior to a long weekend, I dreaded the lack of contact James and I would have because he was also taking an additional vacation day. I wanted to cement myself in his mind so that the four days would not provide relief from me, but instead would keep him full of me so that the following week he would need me even more. I asked him to stop by my office around lunch time while he was running errands. Just to drop in to say hello. He was surprised, knowing that my office would be full of employees and that my family was prone to stopping by unannounced from time to time. I knew Mark was at the gym and would not be likely to drop in. Even though this was more risk that I usually allowed, I really wanted to see him. He seemed very pleased and I knew he would go right to his car and come to me.

I ran off to the gym, making an excuse to ask Mark something to ensure he was in the middle of his workout and would not arrive at my office anytime soon. Now that we had discussed some of what I was going through, it was a safe assumption that he would be paying more attention to my whereabouts.

I rushed back to my office to be there before James arrived. I closed the door after we entered. He looked so good in sleek, taupe slacks and a beautiful short-sleeved print silk shirt showing off his huge shoulders. We reached for each other instinctively, each prior meeting earning us more intimate familiarity. We sat at my conference table, him pulling up my chair close to him so that he could be touching me at all times. I was almost certain that the big picture window behind my desk was reflective enough in its coating that no one from the outside parking lot could see in. I hoped I was right. His hands went immediately to my thighs, telling me once again what beautiful legs I had and how much he wanted to kiss them. Then he reached over to kiss me deeply. I knew how comfortable we were becoming attached in this way. How natural it felt. His hands concentrated on my breasts and my erect nipples popped through my blouse. I closed my eyes, enjoying the sensation completely. He dropped his head deep into my lap, breathing in the smell and feel of me. My organs seemed to disappear, nothing but sensations flying around inside my otherwise hollow body.

As usual, when it was over and time for him to go, he collected himself and moved into his "detach" mode. I could never affect him again after he had made that transition. I often made the mistake of trying.

On that dangerous afternoon in my office, at my insistence, he promised to miss me over the next four days. Then he left. This encounter left me feeling sullen and testy. Because this time I had allowed myself to truly participate, to invest in the experience, holding nothing back. I said under my breath that I had to stop this, then went out to the parking lot to make sure that no one could see into my office through the big picture window. I missed him and wanted him to come back. But mostly I wanted him to think about me the same way I was thinking about him. But I still didn't want to have sex with him.

CHAPTER THIRTY-SIX

Despite my best efforts to inspire Mark to honor the celibacy agreement, we slipped more than once. He didn't take it seriously and seemed to enjoy the rule breaking and I didn't have the will power to refuse him when he wanted me. I continued to enjoy his renewed sexual interest in me.

I tried to behave on our Saturday night dinner out, but towards the end of the evening, I couldn't help sharing with him the overwhelming difficulty of dealing with the emotional residue of my current state of mind. I did not admit my level of involvement with James but did let him know how surprised he would be, perhaps even shocked, by the intensity of my inner life. He knew I was writing a journal, a manuscript, but I saw it only as a medication for the symptoms of my addiction, not a cure. He expressed concern that I was not reaching orgasm regularly and couldn't understand why that would be the case if I was going through such a sexual awakening. I couldn't tell him that my sexual feelings for James caused me so much guilt, affecting my ability to connect with Mark in that way. I explained the importance of the celibacy agreement which allowed me to be free of the feeling that I was putting so much unwanted pressure on him. He apologized and agreed to strict adherence to the agreement. But two days later, on the holiday, we slipped again.

CHAPTER THIRTY-SEVEN

During a terse lunch, James became increasingly surly and sarcastic, feeling that I wasn't making time for him, leaving him frustrated and angry. Who could blame him really? He admitted that I had been different in our office encounter, commenting that the wall I always had around me and that he always bumped into was down and he "went right through me." It was true. I told him how my energy was always so overwhelming that I had learned long ago to control it to protect people. He looked me straight in the eye and said that no matter how much energy I had, he would take all of it, use it up, absorb it like a sponge and not leave me until I was completely spent. My comments about how I liked emotional attachment, and he did not, came out sounding hostile. He said he wanted to leave. And did.

This allowed me to turn once again to my husband for what I wanted and needed, James' hostility an invitation to do so. Mark was feeling very attracted to me, very sexual, but it was impossible to enjoy it completely considering that my response emanated partly from my shameful lust for James.

James became increasingly tense and irritable, sick of waiting for me but unable to call the whole thing off. He could be very mean, which, although hurtful, was actually helpful in shedding light on the utter misery of this hopeless situation. I was overcome by the notion that I was actually putting up with this childish, selfish, immature nonsense from a man when I was married to such a wonderful man who cared about me completely and was incapable of such bad behavior. I wanted to tell my husband everything so badly, but simply could not find the courage. I continued to try to deal with it on my own. My behavior was so inappropriate that I could not even imagine sharing it with anyone for fear of what they would think of me. I knew intellectually that I was wrong and probably why I had the feelings, but I could not actually change the feelings themselves. After my latest nasty encounter with James, which had hurt me badly, I was terribly upset to be out of contact with him and did not know how to cope with the pain and loss. In my head, I knew that this needed to be my cue to make the break, to curb the addiction and learn to do without. But I couldn't stop thinking about him and what he was doing and how he was feeling. I couldn't stop imagining how it would feel to go to him and put all this behind us and get on with what we had to do together.

I felt sick and sad and pathetic and weak. Transparent and empty. Almost as though it was only he who validated my very existence. Without him I couldn't feel the same about myself. It was worse than I could even imagine. What could I do? How could I find my way back?

I would start by not calling him and not accepting his calls if he chose to make contact with me. I wondered if I could.

And yet the very next morning I had changed my plan, vowing not to be victimized and hurt by this man. Instead I would play the game better than he ever dreamed anyone could. And I knew I could, having learned power and control from my father, the master. Even James was not better at this than I was. I vowed to have the last word and turn the tables on him in order to make myself feel better. For the first time in my conscious memory, I thought of hurting him on purpose. I would leave him a message on his voice mail saying that I was sitting in my car in front of a small motel, a little nicer than the dump I had become used to with him, that would be a perfect place for us to meet. Of course I would make the call from my office or my car and I would not be in front of any such motel. Then he would think that I had actually been ready and willing and he had missed it. It would start everything all over again.

What was I thinking? I had absolutely no idea.

CHAPTER THIRTY-EIGHT

I pulled over to the side of the road, prepared to implement my hurtful plan of attack, pulled up the antenna on my cellular phone and dialed his private office number. He answered! Damn. I quickly hung up just as he was beginning to speak. I arrived back at my office two minutes later and found a message that he had just called, practically at the same moment that I had placed my call to him. It unnerved me completely. How could we be so in tune when we were so completely out of touch?

I waited several hours to call back, thinking he was going to apologize for his recent behavior. When we finally spoke, he was in a state that I recognized all too well. He sighed deeply before he even spoke, dark, depressed, and upset. He asked for a "visit" early the following week. I knew it was for the purpose of cutting all contact, saying he wouldn't see me anymore. Even though this had happened before, I was always surprised to recognize how deeply involved he was in all of this and how vulnerable he could be in spite of his serious efforts to the contrary.

Ironically, things were going incredibly well with Mark and I had no intention of jeopardizing that in any way. He finally verbalized to me how much he appreciated the changes I had made, how much less pressure he felt from me. I had been struck by a piece in a woman's magazine about women who were supposedly happily married but were also having affairs. The article was justifying their choices, describing how the affairs could actually improve their marital relationships. One woman said there was nothing more unattractive in a woman than sexual frustration. I agreed with that and had decided to give up sexual neediness with my husband. Partly I thought it was because I knew I could have James anytime and now that I had freely given myself that choice and decided against it, I didn't feel so deprived anymore. I also discovered that the more I backed off from wanting anything sexual from Mark, the more he was drawn to me and my independence. This freed me to express the more loving and sensual parts of myself in a way that we could both enjoy and even seemed to relish lately.

In preparation for my "visit" with James, I had a serious talk with myself. I seemed to be gradually pulling away from this hold he had on me. I forced myself to think about the things that had bothered me about him all along. How controlling he was, how untruthful he could be, how moody he was, how he would become obsessed with his need for me to the exclusion of other conversation or recognition of my life away from him. I reminded myself of how much I had to hold back with him in order to play the game well enough to keep my place in his life. How he would say one thing and then moments later, completely change his position. He simply could not be trusted, ever.

On a deeper and much more painful level, I realized how like my father he was. And to think that I was actually contributing to the pain that he had already caused his wife and daughter. His daughter and I had been friends ever since the day she walked into my dance class. She babysat for us. We shared stories of problems with our fathers so I knew firsthand the challenges she had faced with him. For this indulgence, James had severely chastised me, causing a hurtful argument. He told me that what was between us must remain absolutely private, that his daughter had come to him after our talk asking a lot of questions about our "friendship." I assured him that I would never even hint to his daughter that we were so close but he could not be convinced. I even suggested that he should look to himself and his own behaviors over the years, inadvertently teaching her to be suspicious. This angered him, causing him to snap at me that I should not try to analyze his family in any way.

In my talk with myself, I acknowledged the need to fight against this, like the warrior I had been for so many years in my battle with my father. I knew in my heart that if I allowed James to come between my husband and me, my father would win and all the work would be for naught. My father would be proving that I could not, after all, be free of him the way I said I was. He was the devil in me, and James was the shape and form it took. So in preparation for the "visit," I was trying to toughen up, get ready for the big game. Quietly I believed that I would withstand and prevail. If Mark knew, he would advise me not to attend the meeting. But I knew as strong as my addiction had become that I had to face it head on, and then walk away of my own free will. Not run away in avoidance. There would be no avoidance.

Despite all of this, I tried not to think about what in my heart I knew about James. He, too, was a victim of an abusive upbringing. His daughter had confided in me that he had once been taken along with a sibling on a motor trip by their father who dropped them off in the middle of the desert several hours away and left them there to make it home on their own. He was ten years old. And then there was the sexual abuse by a neighbor woman. He was always suppressing his feelings or trying to meet his needs secretly in situations filled with guilt which he once said could "eat you alive." He was tremendously emotional and, like me, could become physically ill with his desire unfulfilled. We were very much alike in many ways but I saw it as weakness that had to be understood and overcome at all costs and he saw it as a lifestyle that had to be carefully indulged. But we longed to complete the connection. And I felt for him so deeply that it hurt. I loved the emotional frailty in James. It would be so hard to walk away and leave him alone, without me.

CHAPTER THIRTY-NINE

James called with a ridiculous story that his schedule all week would not allow him to meet me for the "visit." Refusing to allow him to have it his way, I bluntly said that it wasn't really his schedule, he was just detaching. He admitted that it was so much easier for him to do this on the phone and then launched right into it. I interjected my irritation that he had told me three days ago that we would meet for this purpose, and now he was changing his mind. I would most certainly prefer doing it in person, finishing it properly. He didn't care. He just wanted to get through it.

On that day, he said many things, most of which were accurate. The energy we had been spending on our counterproductive relationship would be better spent on our own families. That he felt bad all the time, ill even, just as I did. That he did not want to sit in a restaurant as we had done the week before with the feeling that I was just leading him around. That he was about to turn forty-six years old and at one time didn't even think he would be alive at that age, and he wanted to feel good when he woke up in the morning. That I seemed to think that he was the same person he was ten or even eighteen years ago and he wasn't. How we were no different from my sister and her addictive problems that were now controlling her disturbed life. He went on about his religious conflict, how his life needed to be about his relationship with Christ and our relationship had become a serious block to that path.

Then he wandered into the false reality zone, a place I was all too familiar with having been raised by my father. He said he never wanted a physical relationship, that it was I who wanted that. The feeling I had inside of me when he made that incredible comment was exactly the same one I had experienced countless times when my father would state some ridiculous idea that was obviously designed to meet his own perverse need at my expense, never mind its utter disconnect from reality or veracity. I remembered how I always engaged in arguments about those statements, to prove how wrong they were, to defend my position no matter what. But I knew it never worked and would not work here. I had to just let him go on with his carefully constructed scenario. He said that he only wanted to be close to me, not to have physical contact. Experience had already taught me that his only access to intimacy was sexual in nature, making his statement more fantastically unbelievable. I immediately catalogued in my mind how he had taken me to the hotel room to be alone with me, how he had repeatedly touched me, kissed me, caressed me, and talked to me about all the things he wanted to do to me and with me. And how I had used every ounce of willpower to prevent him from getting inside of me, literally. It was I who had hoped to stay close without the sex but he was simply incapable of that.

I assured him that he would get no argument from me in his plan to stop seeing or talking to one another. I fully agreed it was an appropriate step to take. I did, however, strongly disagree with the tone he was using to suggest that I was to blame for all of this and that he was releasing himself from my aggressive pursuit. I suggested that we support one another in this difficult but necessary move and speak honestly in order to help each other deal with the pain we had already experienced and the more intense pain of separation that was sure to follow.

He spoke of how bad our behavior had been, how bad we were for having done it. I would not accept that and suggested that we, instead, say something positive at this moment about our feelings. He said I should go first. Feeling suddenly emotional, and with tears, I explained that I knew that it was all wrong for us to have been as intimate as we had become but that I did not regret a single moment of it. I had needed him, he had taught me many things that I had no other way to learn. I said that I had never done anything like it prior to this time with him and would never again. But it was right and important for me and I had a place for him that would never be relinquished to anyone else, and I was not sorry. I said that with the unbelievably intense connection between us, we had shown each other and our families tremendous respect by not taking it much further than we had. We, in fact, should be proud that we had exerted as much self-control as we had.

When it was his turn, he very quietly and with much effort said that the kindness and friendship that I had shown him had meant so much to him. That his heart was still full of anger and hurt and pain and that I had eased that pain, gotten through to him and made a difference. And that was the part he would take with him. And that he cared about me so much. But we simply couldn't go on this way.

I asked him to help me understand just how we were going to do it. He said he would do it one hour at a time. Then he wondered how we should end this conversation. Determined that this time, I would be the one to go first, I said good-bye and hung up the phone.

I thought there was something different about this parting, even though there had been others that had seemed equally traumatic at the time. It seemed more permanent somehow. I was grateful that he had found the courage to do it because I knew I could never find it in myself. I just wanted to ride the wave until it broke. But at that moment, I was devastated and terrified, wondering how I could ever give him up. I was numb. My pride would not allow me to go to him after that conversation but I still wanted to. I wanted him to hold me, kiss me, comfort me, and make me feel all those feelings. I couldn't imagine a time when I would not want that from him.

Having no idea how this could ever work for me, I went home and went straight to my room, lying still on my bed. Then I went to the dance studio, which had increasingly become my haven. Later, I awoke in the middle of the night, panic-stricken over what had happened. No, I could definitely not do this.

The following morning I became partially hysterical with Mark, crying and curling up in a ball. He wondered aloud what could have done this to me and I wouldn't say but tried to cover it with details of my concern over my sister and her deepening struggles. I asked him to call the therapist I had been seeing and try to get me an appointment. That made me feel better and as I lay there on the bed, he began to touch me and treat me in a sexual way. I knew that he really wanted me at that moment and it made me very happy and I gave myself to him. This was a wonderful thing for me, a sign of hope, a place to go from where I was.

James had told me that we should go back to where we had come from. I emphatically said that I would never go back to where I had come from. That instead I would make a new life with what I had learned. Now I brought those lessons to my marriage. And it was a real breakthrough. It was amazing to me how I had been able to manage amidst all the turmoil. And that Mark was smart and secure enough to see that I needed complete space and privacy in which to work all this out. I could not imagine another living man who could have given me that.

I had a wonderful session with my therapist. He helped me see this as a positive step and an opportunity for me to continue on in my healing journey. He promised me that I would gradually become more and more comfortable and happy in that golden aura I had seen around Mark that day I returned from the dreadful motel encounter. That it would resonate to me and it would fill that empty space inside me. That I should think in terms of energy and ride my excellent instincts. He always helped me clean out the toxic feelings and get back to myself. When I asked for help as to how to ride out the withdrawal from my addiction to James, he said simply to "let it slide." He urged me to remember that it was my choice, that I could simply choose. I was filled with hope.

On the way home, I stopped by our neighborhood clubhouse where Andrew was working, Mark was working out, and Peter was playing pool by himself. Mark expressed genuine concern as to my state of mind, Andrew told me how the maintenance man thought I must be his sister because I looked so young, and I played pool with Peter and enjoyed it more than I could ever imagine. I realized how long it had been since I had been able to do that. I let the three of them fill me up and hold me tight and I basked in the joy it gave me.

CHAPTER FORTY

I attended a presentation by Marilyn Van Derbur, former Miss America, about her experience with paternal sexual abuse. Start with a bucket of white paint, she said, and then add red paint to it. There is no part of the original white paint that is not impacted by adding the red. That is sexual abuse. It colors everything. Every single part of your life thereafter.

My red paint consisted of the obvious influence of my father's sexual view of the world, my mother's permanent victim status and inability to protect us, my sister's lifelong battles with coming to terms with what happened to her, and now my own need to jeopardize everything that mattered to me with proof that I belonged to my father's legacy. The red paint seeped its way into my soul and my existence and my sense of myself until I no longer recognized my own face in the mirror.

It prevented me from seeing that my marriage, in the sexual sense, was vital and spontaneous and passionate and loving and respectful. But all I valued was the extreme and obsessive sexual connection to a man who was as addicted to our secret relationship as I was. And no one else could compete with that.

As a child, when our home began to sink into its terrible state of abuse, I managed to instinctively collect the very essence of what I knew to be goodness in me and lock it away in a golden box inside. What I didn't know was if it would ever be safe to retrieve it. I believe that it was the hope in the sweet, innocent contents of that box that kept me from consummating my relationship with James in the face of unbearable pressure to do so, trying with all my heart to avoid complete irreversible immersion into the darkness of sexual abuse.

I went to see the therapist who had originally treated my sister when her life began to unravel and who later treated my parents at the time when my father revealed his lifelong pattern of infidelity. I knew that the doctor was sympathetic to my mother who had not at that time, and has still not, recognized her own victim status. What made me want to work with him was his knowledge of my family and its dynamics. That would not only save me hours of time in therapy, but would help to validate the enormous difficulties of trying to survive my particular extended family. He pointed out that it might be inappropriate for him to treat both my parents and me, that it could be perceived as a conflict of interest. I said I understood but convinced him that we could work together without breaking his patient confidentiality. He agreed. Somehow it was easier to confide in him the double life I was leading because knowing where I came from, I felt he would be less likely to judge me as the terrible person I thought myself to be by this time. I began seeing him on a regular basis, trying to keep my head above water as abuse continually tried to pull me under the surface. He was able to confirm the many conclusions I was forming about my family history and its impact on my current situation while still honoring his commitment to my parents in their own therapy.

I continued to write in painstaking detail about what was happening to me. That process helped me hold on to the good in my life. Somehow I could see the enormity of the risk associated with my choices by writing about them and then reading the words. It was a very painful process as I had never in my life experienced feelings and urges that simply could not be controlled. It was very hard for me to understand why my behavior could not be stopped as a matter of will. Mark recognized it all and had grave concerns, somehow knowing that he could not make demands or speed up the process because what seemed so obvious to him was not yet known to me. I will always be grateful for his wisdom in allowing me to continue down the road, all the while knowing what it might cost him, our family and me.

On more than one occasion, Mark warned me that if I were not careful, I would make a tumor to house the stress that had taken over my physical and psychological life. He knew that I was fully capable of such a thing. Even though he sometimes said it in a lighthearted way, it had an ominous tone to it and I knew there was truth in it. Actually, finding a way to collect all the stress into any one receptacle seemed appealing to me. At least it wouldn't be swirling around like drops of red paint dripping into the bucket of white.

CHAPTER FORTY-ONE

The immediate sensation of peace and relief that followed the phone "visit" with James disappeared in short order and was replaced by plans and schemes to get him back. Despite various unsuccessful attempts to see him and call him during the first week, I managed to survive.

The following week, I was still planning a visit to discuss the importance of our long, enduring friendship and how it should be preserved at all costs. But I was choosing my wardrobe carefully for just the right effect. He should not be allowed to believe that I would accept what he said, and rudely at that. I would do as I pleased just to show him I could. If I wanted a "visit," I could have one. After all that mental exercise, I still didn't call, probably because I had proved to myself that I could if I wanted. So I didn't need to.

Gradually, thoughts of him lessened and I began to feel strangely calm and composed, more open to sexual play with Mark that didn't have the undercurrent of deception. Days passed and I felt stronger. I convinced myself that I hadn't felt this "well" in years, that now it was time to test my progress.

I accepted a lunch date with a colleague of James' in an adjacent building to his office. So almost casually, I called his private line to let him know I would be on campus and could drop by for a visit. He answered in a good mood and was receptive and relaxed.

He readily agreed. I made a point of saying it would be after my luncheon, knowing he would be jealous. I felt that surge of power return, knowing I had affected him in exactly the way I had planned.

The lunch took longer than expected so I arrived late. I was shocked to see him looking so grim, pale yet dark, and emotionally exhausted. I could see that he had not managed the past nine days as well as I had. If he had been doing well, he would not have allowed the visit at all. I tried not to allow his pain to get to me and prepared to proceed with my rehearsed lines, struggling to show him how positive and resigned I was to our new arrangement.

He immediately questioned me as to why I was late, pushing for details of the lunch. As predicted, he was irritated that I made time for my lunch partner but not for him so many times in the past.

I continued with my statement, saying I was there for two reasons. The first was to tell him of a very real, intense dream I had about him that was so disturbing that I wanted to make sure for myself that he was okay. He wanted to hear about it.

I was in my office meeting with a man and a woman but for some reason my office looked exactly like James' instead. I told the two visitors that they could stay but that I was expecting another guest any moment. They said fine and continued on with their business. James arrived looking awful, dressed sloppily in sweat clothes with old, saggy socks and beat up tennis shoes. His posture was slumped and sagging. His appearance was in complete contrast to his usual strong, neat and powerful presence. I was shocked to see him looking that way and as he sat down in the old grey chair in front of the desk, I instinctively went to him. He grabbed me by the waist and pulled me down into his lap and I did not resist. I began rubbing his shoulders trying to help him regain his posture. Strangely, the other man in the room whipped out a small remote control device and began making the chair spin, slowly at first and then faster and faster until we were spinning completely out of control, clutching each other tightly. Then I awoke.

He listened intently to my dream and then smiled, saying that he supposed that was one for the therapist to ponder. But I knew he was completely aware of the obvious symbolism of the dream.

My second reason for visiting was to acknowledge my respect for our original friendship which I believed to be intact, even after all we had been through. I didn't know if it could find shape and form between us, but I wanted him to know that it still existed for me and how much I valued it. He said it took time. He went on to say how hurtful it could have all become and how overcome he was with intuitive fear toward the end.

Throughout the visit, I felt his eyes looking through me, filled with desire that was not only physical. He was struggling to repeat all the proper reasons for our separation but the need was still very much present. The question was how would I respond to being subjected to it again? I reminisced about our first meeting when I was seventeen years old and my perfect plan that he would ask me out, pick me up at the door, and deliver me back there after our date. How when I discovered that he was married, I knew we could never have that. And now I had a family of my own. I reminded him that we had always agreed that we would not change our lives to be together. He looked away in obvious distress. Was it possible that he still entertained such a notion?

His secretary alerted him that his next appointment had arrived, so I took that as my cue to leave. I had accomplished what I came for, on my own terms and felt I could find more peace in the outcome now rather than feeling controlled and enraged by the terms he had placed on all of this just nine days ago.

I did not feel the old overpowering urge to go back to him the rest of the day. I had passed the test.

CHAPTER FORTY-TWO

There were a few days when I did not even think about sex and did not miss thinking about it. Periods of time actually passed when I did not think about James at all. I was more able to share my energy with co-workers, my children and my husband.

But then there were moments where I found myself practicing how I was going to ask James to run away with me, my hand already on the phone. There were deep, strong fantasies that I knew could become reality. But I continued to choose sanity, honesty, respect, sacrifice and self-esteem. It was the hardest thing I had ever tried to do. And it required an effort every moment of every day. What was I supposed to do with those incredibly intense feelings? I assumed I would probably just have to forego the process of uncovering my deepest sexual identity. Was it too much to give up? I didn't know.

CHAPTER FORTY-THREE

Mark and I began to struggle. He would ask for space and distance himself from me which would simply enhance my desire to run to the man who wanted anything but distance from me. Mark tried to understand the intensity of my needs and said that if the way we lived together was so foreign to me, so against my nature, then maybe I should try to find a life that was more accommodating. At least I might want to spend some time apart to explore those feelings on my own. Then I could come back and report on my findings. I asked what might happen if I found I did not want that life. He wasn't sure. It never dawned on me that he might just not want to struggle with me anymore, but I could see he had actually entertained the idea. The very fact that we were having this conversation suggested that the isolation from James was affecting my marriage negatively. Even though I had not been sleeping with him, I had been getting so much sexual attention from him and now I was certain my husband was feeling all that pressure coming back on him. My emotional panic must have been easy to read.

Feeling lost and confused, I dressed for the dance studio. Before I left, Mark pulled me to his lap, holding me tightly. Our deep love and affection for each other overcame the tremendous pain of the recent past. I walked away, not expecting anything to progress, but he followed me to the kitchen and pressed against me, kissing me deeply, hands roaming over my dance clothes. He seemed overwhelmed with passion for me, lifting me off the floor to accommodate the foot difference in our height, holding me tight. He swept me up in his arms and carried me upstairs to our bed. He made love to me in a way he never had before, resulting in the deepest orgasm I had ever had, causing me to nearly lose consciousness. I was so overcome that I burst into tears and sobbed uncontrollably. All this time I felt that I couldn't affect my husband in this way, and yet he seemed deeply affected. Still something prevented me from believing and accepting that.

I felt completely well, spiritually at rest, more content than I could ever imagine.

CHAPTER FORTY-FOUR

My journal continued to reflect my conflict and the comings and goings of my emotional state. The only thing that gave me a break was my annual vacation to the shore in the summer. Looking out the ceiling to floor windows of the small condo we rented every year on the eighth floor, I could see nothing but sea and sky. My long walks took me down an isolated stretch of Navy beach where I would stop for dance exercises in the sand, face the ocean and let the breeze caress me as I moved and stretched and breathed and existed under the sky in front of the waves. This ritual had a powerful healing effect on me.

Mark was more than willing to have sex with me but it was clear that I was getting something out of it that had nothing to do with him, working through something, and he began calling me a monster. I missed James, who didn't characterize me in that way, who loved my voraciousness and found it irresistible.

One morning, very early, I thought I was dreaming. It was still dark and something drew me to the window. On the beach below, men were setting up luminaries and torches in a path as though preparing for some type of ritual. As the sun rose, I realized it was a Mexican wedding. A woman began to play the harp. Soon a young barefoot Mexican woman in a white dress married a small white man in a suit that he was lost in. It was a dream of marriage. I thought of the ritual as a birth and a death. Sometimes I felt dead inside, longing for something more.

Two and a half weeks had passed since any contact with James. I was sure he was sticking to his plan to let me go. I had come a long way towards accepting that during my stay at the shore. The tranquility and simple familiarity of life there was like medicine. The long walks with the ocean breeze served to clean out my troubled soul. I had also noticed that my physical cravings had begun to diminish to what I imagined to be a normal level. Mark and I were enjoying each other regularly and fully and I was feeling satisfied.

When calling my office to check messages, I was stunned to discover that the receptionist was actually on a line with a call for me and asked if I could wait a moment. It was James, his second call of the day. He wanted to know if I had returned, explaining in the message that he was leaving town for two weeks himself, apparently on the very day I was to arrive back home. I knew this meant that as he was preparing to leave, he needed to connect with me. I felt the usual surge of energy because truthfully I hated the times when we were trying to give each other up.

I decided it was far too risky to return that call, allowing that part of my life to infringe on my clean, healthy, idyllic family beach time. No, I definitely wouldn't risk that, I thought, as I put my hand to the phone and dialed his private line.

He said he had hoped I was back and could see him before he left town. I not only allowed the conversation to go where it shouldn't have, I initiated it. He admitted that he was taking their separation one day at a time now, considering it an improvement over the original one hour at a time method. We talked of seeking opportunities in the future, I wished him a safe journey, he detached and it was over.

I felt deflated that I had allowed this phone interlude to take place and in some ways, the residue was surprisingly unwelcome.

But I didn't feel guilty about it and had a wonderful evening with Mark anyway. He informed me that despite that look in my eye, we would not have sex until the morning. I seduced him anyway and he seemed to like that. We were happy. I would just have to work the other thing out somehow.

CHAPTER FORTY-FIVE

My two weeks back at the office were filled with stress and I could not wait to get back to the shore. James was on his vacation so we were completely out of touch. When he returned, I would be going back to California. It was a very long break for us.

A close friend's mother died suddenly and I made plans to go back for the day to attend the funeral. James had called asking if I had returned yet, knowing full well I had not, but asking for a return call anyway. I knew that if I went home for the day, I could call him and maybe see him. And I did.

He came to my office and then gave me a ride to the airport. Our reunion and the passionate turn it took caused me to almost miss my flight. He begged me to stay overnight and spend it with him, burying his head in my breasts. I, of course, made him take me to the airport.

And so I fell off the wagon just as sure as if I had been my sister taking a drink. I had been solid and calm for the many weeks of our separation. But now, the game was back on. Maybe later I could figure out how I should be handling all of this. But not now. Definitely not now. Not yet.

I planned to see James again upon my return, feeling ready to go right back to his arms. But I could not reach him. Not for a week. Then he called saying he had been sent out of town on business, sweet in his tone. I was to call him after a court appearance that afternoon. Things went very badly in court. He heard it in my voice, asked me about it, then retracted the question saying it would take too long for me to explain. He insensitively said something about losing some and winning some. Then he said it was late and asked me not to stop by, even though I was almost there by that time. The combination of a totally unjust verdict against me and his cold insensitivity was very hard to take. He had always told me not to depend on him. He was proving that he meant it.

The next day we spoke on the phone, a call I initiated. He instructed me to close the door, which I did, and proceeded to put on the James phone sex show, completely detached, servicing me. He didn't follow through on a possible plan to stop by later. But I went to him the next day. He didn't kiss me. Mostly he was interested in my crotch. He was more detached than ever before, as if his feelings were no longer involved and he could no longer get hurt. And I couldn't have hurt more.

CHAPTER FORTY-SIX

I delivered another chapter of my manuscript to James, which so honestly expressed my emotions that, as I hoped, it opened him up and gave me access to him once again. He gave me the answer I was looking for and it brought tears to my eyes. Warm, wonderful, painful, relief filled tears.

He visited me, to talk this time. He spoke of how he had just cried one day over his constant and lifelong goal to become the person he hoped to be, wanted to be more than anything else. He wanted to be honest and true and good and right. He believed he had made real progress towards that goal but his feelings for me produced deep conflict. I understood that his occasional detachment and anger were really the embodiment of that conflict. He spoke of self-destructive behavior, including what we did in his office, saying that he had lived that life for years and didn't wish to revisit it. But he admitted that his feelings for me were not just physical, that he also loved who I was, what I did, how I said things. It was everything. But he also admired my goodness, my choices, my commitment to my family. He did not wish to be responsible for disturbing that. I added that I did not wish to be associated in his mind with the strong negative self-image of his past. Nothing would be worth that. He seemed relieved to hear me say that, his eyes filling with tears. He gradually moved back from me in his chair until distance was created between us. He looked so vulnerable and I knew how exposed he must have been feeling. I loved him for his rare honesty at that moment and it gave me peace and understanding to connect in this way. I had always believed that he did not want to hurt me, even though he was totally capable of that. He had given me sexual self-esteem, a sensual awareness of myself, the feeling of beauty and feminine power, the sense of being completely desired, the choices. . . all things I had missed along the way. Gently, sweetly, safely, but completely all the same.

When he left, he held me and kissed me and begged me to allow him to bring me to an orgasm. He wanted to do that for me and it was important to him. But not on this day, not there in my office.

And so he gave me the gift of letting me go, not making me go through with it, and making me feel okay about it. He did not run away saying that we could never see each other again. He left it wide open, no decisions, each of us wondering if there would ever be a time when we could come together without sacrificing ourselves too much.

I felt intense emotional relief upon his departure. I had incredibly strong feelings for him, believing that God had sent him to protect me while still giving me every single experience necessary to overcome my past and hopefully save my future.

My parents came to the beach to sign the sale papers for my purchase of the company. It wasn't what they wanted but they knew they had no choice. At that moment, when I officially took control of what used to be theirs, I thought it might be safe to crack open the golden box inside of me. It just might be safe enough to consider letting myself out.

CHAPTER FORTY-SEVEN

Once again I found myself in a motel room with James, a different dump this time. It wasn't planned but I went willingly. For the first time I allowed him to put his head between my legs although I wouldn't remove my pantyhose and stopped short of a climax for the same reason as all the other times. I found that once I was in position, literally, I didn't want to, couldn't bear to.

He was used to that but this time wanted me to do the same for him, gently pushing my head down, complaining that I never touched him there, where he wanted it the most. I wouldn't, but couldn't help noticing that even with all this going on, he was not erect. I felt confused and disappointed by this. He spoke of teaching me how to stimulate him while I was busy wondering why he wasn't already stimulated. I did not wish to be taught to do anything of the sort.

I proudly showed him how I had let my nails grow longer and had put clear polish on them so they looked nice. He was not the least bit interested when I explained that I was tired of his nails looking more manicured than mine. He was so frustrated with me and had only one thing on his mind. And it was not my nails.

I smelled like him on my hands, in my hair and all over my body. I was soaked through my pantyhose. Back at my office, I went to the bathroom and with a wet paper towel, washed between my legs. I really, really didn't want this.

In the next few days, I began to feel a heavy, vague discomfort between my legs. I snuck off to Urgent Care to be examined. The doctor questioned my sexual practices, whether I had multiple partners, mentioning the possibility of chlamydia. He instructed me to stop wearing underwear for a few days and let things "air out." I told him I was married, completely monogamous, and had made the mistake of wearing pantyhose without underwear. He seemed skeptical but sent me on my way with no diagnosis. I was horrified that my miserable experience in the motel room could have led to this equally miserable trip to the doctor. I avoided sex with Mark, terrified that maybe I had become infected with something. I couldn't bear the thought of passing it on to him. But I wanted him to make love to me. If only I could get through this part, I felt I could go to him completely.

Things improved with my symptoms and I waited patiently until Mark came to me, asking if we could meet at home over lunch to play together. I was as happy as could be. Overjoyed, totally satisfied.

When James called, I told him about my trip to the doctor. He assured me he was a blood donor and was quite sure he could not have been the cause of my problem. I mentioned my stockings and he couldn't help mentioning how I kept them on for dear life. Things turned very serious as he told me how difficult it had been for him since that day. He had been physically ill, tormented by the combination of sexual frustration and how wrong he knew it was for us to be together that way. He had been to his priest who had advised him that the only way to deal with all of it was to completely eliminate me from his life. And he was taking the next three days off to go up north to an isolated cabin alone in order to think about things. Or perhaps he would just serve food to people who didn't have enough to eat. He was feeling pretty bad about himself. He cried more than once during the talk and said that I was the only part of his life that was not what he wanted it to be. He asked me not to call when he was back. I agreed and said I understood everything. I told him I loved him. He said he knew, and amazingly it was I who detached this time.

My discomfort did not go away on its own. I was examined again at Urgent Care, this time with my husband along. The doctor again questioned my sex life, mentioning chlamydia. I wanted to ask if it could be spread by oral contact but couldn't bring myself to do it. He prescribed an antibiotic.

I was so fearful that my behavior had caused this terrible outbreak of a sexually transmitted disease even though I had not had intercourse. I played over and over in my mind what we had done in an effort to determine if it was possible. I read up on everything I could find. I was ashamed and sick that I had to keep these fears from Mark. I did share, in tears, how upsetting it was for the doctor to question me that way. He laughed and said it didn't matter since I told him I was married and wasn't sexual with anyone else. He didn't understand, but how could he? The heaviness in my bladder was a constant reminder of what I had done and I was convinced in my mind that I was being punished. I promised myself that I had learned my lesson and that I would never engage in such behavior again, begging God to let me have one more chance.

At 4 am one morning, I found myself at the computer writing a letter to James that, of course, I would never send. It just seemed important to say it "to" him, rather than "about" him as I did in my journal.

Dear James,

I feel angry. Thank God. We have had very little contact since the day at the motel where you put your head between my legs. And all of that contact has been controlled by you. You have detached in order to protect yourself. But you can't let go because you haven't finished. The explosion, the surge, the resolution is not yet yours.

You did not realize how very right you were when you said that I was more like you than you first imagined. You have been, strangely, angel and devil to me. After having controlled my feelings so perfectly for so long, when I let them out it was you who nudged them awake and gave them life. The angel in you allowed me to feel all those wonderful sexual feelings without asking me to compromise on the things that are the most important in the world to me. The devil in you doesn't care about me at all. You try to control my behavior, meet your needs, and move on to how much easier it was when you did not have to deal with me. You try to have it both ways but it doesn't work with me. You let me know that you do not wish to waste time in any activity that does not directly lead to the explosion, the surge, the resolution.

But I am not that incensed after all. I was duly hurt when you were curt with me on the phone. And when you finally opened that door again by suggesting that I recreate the environment where we could "finish," it got to me. When I got home that night, it was unusual that no one was there. I began undressing. As I did, I became aware of my body. I began to enjoy undressing, thinking about you. I left on only my high heels, black. And I took a good long look in the mirror. I liked the way I looked. I wondered, not for the first time, why I had never taken my clothes off for you, never given myself or you that pleasure. And I vowed that I would never go to a private room with you again unless I was prepared to take all of my clothes off. I put my own hand between my legs and took a long time bringing myself to a very nice orgasm. An explosion, a surge, a resolution. For a few days, I could feel you, your hands on me, your lips, your head between my legs. And I liked it very much.

And since the other day in the motel, I have had more contact than usual with other men. I have played golf with two different groups. And I have lunched or met with no less than seven men. This is not a coincidence. It takes a lot of men to replace you. And none of them do, by the way.

But back to my anger. You have taken all the joy, all of the friendship, and reduced it to the surge, the explosion, the resolution. You are almost ready to detach completely, but there is that damned unfinished business.

The part that is so difficult for me is the connection to my father. He prepared me all my life for my relationship with you. He told me how it was going to be. That you would always want the sex. That it would always control things. That you would not want it after you got it. That it was a supreme source of power. That it was everything. But I feel strangely at home in my soul with you, in the most terrifying way. Just like Dad said. Every single thing about him that I rejected out of disgust, I later found in you. It was inevitable. And I hate that part of him. And I love and hate that part of you. Love it because it makes me feel that I have succeeded, that I can play the game I was taught so well, and that I am a real woman in my father's eyes. Hate it because it is so damned destructive. And hate it because I love it.

But I swear underneath all of that behavior, which I understand and relate to so well, I love who you are. I love touching that part of you, finding it intact every now and then. When you are honest with me, when you trust me, when your eyes fill with tears as mine have now. I love that part so much, and I believe in it, in its goodness, and its hope and its joy so much that I have trouble staying angry and even more trouble letting go. Because I suppose I am afraid that if I let you go, that part of you will go with it. When actually, my God, letting you go will probably give even more life to that wonderful part of you. I just won't be a part of it.

It is no wonder I suffer so when you tell me how bad we are for what we have done, how wrong it is, and then tell me later how we should do it some more. But the suffering is the thing after all. I didn't understand it while it was buried under all those layers of protection. When I shed the layers, I suffered more than I thought possible. You have always understood that and every time we have touched, it has eased the suffering. Not like sex really. Just so intimate, so powerful, providing so much instantaneous relief. Thus the addiction. But don't all addicts think that their alcohol or drug use is easing their pain and suffering? When really, it has caused more suffering than it will ever be able to ease.

But I am angry. Angry that you think so little of me. I have spent a lifetime trying to prove my father wrong and trying to believe in the things that are right and good. Why and how I let you reduce me to a place to finish; the explosion, the surge, the resolution. When you won't even be in the room.

And, no, it was obviously not safe to begin to explore the contents of the golden box inside.

CHAPTER FORTY-EIGHT

Ihad neglected to notice during all this time that while I was obsessed with trying to survive my illicit obsession with James, my husband had begun to change in very significant ways.

He reached out for me in the car, between my legs, talking about how we would make love later. He teased me about my fantasies, my constant sexual readiness, and seemed to accept this part of me in a loving and affectionate way. He opened himself physically to me in a new way. I couldn't wait to get home to him in the evening, to see a movie with him knowing he would see it in exactly the same way that I did. He seemed proud of how I had worked out my problems, knowing how difficult it was.

One evening over dinner, I told him how much it meant to me that he had let me go when I needed him to even though it was so scary. How there was no other man in the world who could have allowed what he did and how it had opened the door to my own feelings and understanding them and choosing for myself. And now I could give myself to him completely, knowing I had everything I wanted, appreciating him in the way he had always deserved to be appreciated. He seemed pleased to be acknowledged in that way.

I slipped off my shoes under the table and stretched my legs out to his side of the booth, placing my bare feet between his knees. He reached down and rubbed my feet, sliding his hands up and down my legs. I placed my hands on the table between us, reaching out to him, and he commented on how beautiful my nails looked.

When we went home and went to bed, he pulled me close and said, "We're in love, aren't we?" I answered yes and drifted off to sleep.

I had truly saved myself. Or so I thought.

CHAPTER FORTY-NINE

It seemed that there was no place left for my relationship with James to go. I had tried doing it, not doing it, seeing him, not seeing him, and finally I hit the wall. I no longer wrote all the searing details in my journal. Somehow not writing it made it seem less real and I talked myself into believing it had run its course and with lessons learned, I was lucky to get out of it intact. But I wasn't intact at all.

I collected my journal into a manuscript which helped make sense of things, giving me a false sense of distance, as though it were someone else's story and had never actually happened to me. I wrote to Mark in the early fall, trying to nudge him closer to the truth:

I have not been well in the past four years, emotionally not well at all. By finishing my manuscript, I have put an end to that part of my life. It is a very scary feeling though to lose that outlet. To know that there is nowhere else to go with it now. That instead, I have to go on without it. I don't even know how to do that. The power and thrill of that intimacy, although not physical in any way, was staggering and spoke very much to the way I had been raised to believe that it should feel. In fact, it fit all the requirements. It was secret, it was profoundly sexual in its nature, it was about control, and I seemed to have the effect on this man that I felt I never had on you. And this was the effect I had long been taught was my birthright. And I seemed to be pretty good at it. It was impossible to turn away. It simply could not be skipped or avoided. I wasn't strong enough for that.

But the enormous energy I put forth over the past four years to keep this under control and still experience it as completely as possible is astounding to me. I am totally exhausted by it, often ashamed of it, and trying hard to forgive myself. Sometimes it is not easy. I perceived it in the beginning to be exercising my right to free choice, to controlling my own world for a change. But somewhere along the line, it began to control me and was as true an addiction as my sister's drinking. I felt powerless to let go of it, but uniquely, in my case, powerless to indulge in it either. My biggest fear was becoming my father so I fought that with all my heart, but inside I felt a lot like him. Still do sometimes. It is astounding how you can get used to almost anything though. Just the sheer repetition made it easier, numbing the shock and horror you feel the first time. In all cases, I could not wait to get back to you and prayed that I had not caused any irreparable damage. I believed in my heart that you would forgive me because you are so strong and smart. I can no longer stand having any of this between us. I pray to God that is because I am seeing so much more clearly now and things that most certainly should have upset me in the past and did not are now plenty upsetting. For that I am grateful. I have absolutely no desire to revisit that place, to experiment, or to continue with this behavior in any way. I love you so much, in a way I could never even feel or understand before. Please forgive me.

I found the nerve to send the manuscript to a man I knew who lived far away, whom I considered a friend. He very much wanted to read it but I was reluctant to reveal the subject matter. It didn't seem to scare him so I took the plunge. It was terrifying and wonderful to release the work to the outside, one more step in releasing it from inside of myself where it had lived alone for so long.

When we arranged a time to discuss it on the phone, his attempts at objective criticism quickly turned into a personal, open and sometimes strangely intimate talk about sex and each of our stories. He had one of his own, to my surprise. The relief of being able to speak openly about my experience with someone I trusted and who would not judge me was overwhelming. He said that my husband was a lucky man, making an offhand remark about how his wife was not always so willing and how aroused he had become as he read my words on a plane. I had never considered, not for one moment, that Mark might be a lucky man. It was like the part of my sexual self-esteem that was still missing came rushing into my heart. Maybe it was true.

I couldn't wait to come home and tell Mark about what my friend had said. It made me feel different, like maybe my feelings were not really an affliction, but a blessing in a new life where I was beginning to integrate myself into one woman. That one man's opinion gave me a new perspective, which I loved and clung to.

It also gave me the opportunity to share with Mark more openly how frustrated I was sometimes, how hard I had worked to access this new part of myself, and how I had risked too much to just put it away now. I told him that my feelings seemed new and needed to be realized. He reminded me that he was a man in his mid-forties who had been in a relationship with the same woman for twenty-two years. He understood what I was saying but did not share my enthusiasm for the journey of discovery I was seeking.

But after that, things changed unexpectedly. He came to me, over and over. I did not initiate sex; he always did. He had never been a stronger or more affectionate, more passionate lover. I continued to grow into myself with this new confidence, feeling stronger and more secure every day.

I thought of James less and less and could not even imagine being intimate with him like I had been for so long. I was grateful for the long space between us and for the fact that he was not calling. When he finally did, I allowed him to speak to me sexually, describing his longing for me, but it was different. I allowed it to wash over me so that I could thoroughly feel that I was no longer affected in the same way, no longer controlled by the longing. My body betrayed my spirit though and I felt the strong physical response, that emptiness that allowed me to imagine only him inside of me and nothing else, not even organs. But I was not ashamed of that. I did not wish to go back to shame, guilt or remorse. Instead I was determined that my sexuality would be a source of love and joy and enrichment, just as it had now become with Mark. I could feel the door behind which James was standing, close.

I felt free in a way I had never known. There was a peace and contentment in this revelation that seemed almost mystical. The edge that I had always carried within myself was gone. I no longer needed to be a warrior, to protect myself at all costs, to control things. I surrendered in victory.

CHAPTER FIFTY

Becoming involved with James was like slowly falling down a dark hole. Sometimes the plunge was exhilarating even though I knew there was nowhere to go but down. I prayed for my fall to be broken by the proverbial rock bottom so I could start the hard climb out, but at the same time, I didn't want the journey to end. And it was always really dark in there.

If all journeys begin at ground level, then getting involved with Michael again was an ascension of the spirit, not a descent of the flesh. He was such a tender soul, so quiet and patient and resolute in his care for me. It seemed perfectly natural for him to reconnect to me because he had continued to nurture that connection for the years we were out of touch. And I could feel that. It had a sense of being old and familiar and already fully formed, ready to be explored further, brought to a higher level, but with a firm foundation. And it was built on trust, already earned long ago.

I was ignorant of how powerful it would become at first because after my years of experience with James, I assumed that someone who lived three thousand miles away could not possibly find his way so deep inside of me. What I didn't know was that in time, our ability to communicate and experience each other did not require that we be in the same physical place. In fact, on the infrequent occasions when we would have a visit, it seemed almost ordinary and anti-climactic as we were mindful to respect our families and ensure that we did not taint our feelings with guilt or shame. Michael saw to that. No matter what his personal desires were, he was very much our leader in terms of keeping things clean. I don't know if it was harder for me or not. I just know he was a lot better at it than I was. And I relied on him for that.

I didn't tell him about the sexual abuse until we had passed a few letters between us and I began to feel more comfortable settling in with our renewed friendship. My frequent letters to Michael replaced my daily journal, my sex log. When fax machines came into our lives, it became a more immediate way to communicate. It was as natural as could be for me to write everything down and send it to him, my most intimate thoughts and feelings. But it came harder to him. He got better at it as he went along and began to succumb to his own feelings rather than just accommodating mine, which he did brilliantly.

He was an artist in every way. He wrote like one, thought like one and painted like one. Even his handwriting was beautiful and lyrical. He had the soul of an artist. I wasn't in love with him, but I came to love him intensely. He cherished me in a way that my parents did not and should have.

Even though I had the joy of being cherished by Mark and my two sons, I was still leading two separate lives. I existed at home in one emotional place but the part of me that was still struggling to find my way out of the powerful and dark impact of abuse was becoming more and more detached from reality. Michael was a place of light for me, where I could exist in warmth and comfort. He was a safe haven that I desperately needed. My letters to him were laced with references to Mr. Arizona, his name for James. I wrote of my constant struggle and confessed when I slipped and did something I shouldn't have. He never judged me harshly but worried about me constantly.

I have only vague memories of my continuing difficult and disappointing experiences with James during this time. Going back to that behavior after believing that I had ended that part of my life was so disturbing that I became better and better at disassociating myself from it, compartmentalizing it more and more. Almost like an out of body experience that had everything to do with my body. There was virtually nothing positive left between us, just a raw need to finish what we started so long ago. He had already established that it was bad for us and we shouldn't be doing it. I had already established that it was highly unlikely that I was ever going to do it anyway. But we couldn't stop. Or wouldn't.

I continued to write to Michael about everything, almost like trying to catch him up on who I had become since we were kids in high school.

I carefully placed safety barriers up around my emotional core for many years as a means of protecting and preserving myself, a natural survival instinct. I forced myself to super achieve, expecting perfection, thus earning my family nickname of Patti Perfect. I did not allow myself free choice or to feel things too deeply as it was too risky. My choices had to be beyond reproach, no mistakes. I chose my husband because he was totally trustworthy (still is), showed me tremendous respect, would never hurt me (and never has), and understood that the environment from which I emerged had profoundly affected my development. He validated my feelings, encouraged me to grow and change separate from my family influences, and was always there to support and encourage during the process. It was also necessary that the man I chose be possessed of true logic and intellect, not driven by personal needs and feelings. Strong and true. Non-threatening. I knew the children I would have with him would be beautiful and strong and would not face the difficulties I had been forced to endure. The woman he met and stayed with, however, is not the woman I am today. Once I moved through this process, I began to get in touch with my warmer, more affectionate, more emotional, more feeling oriented self which is who I honestly believe I would have been from the beginning if it had been safe. I removed a lot of the controls I had in place up until that time and probably went off the deep end in a way. What a shock it has been for my poor husband. So I struggle to put a lid on what feels like a tidal wave of emotion which has been safely hidden inside me for so many years, thinking this lid will allow me to continue to fit into my own life. But the lid keeps popping off and the truth is that I worked so damned hard to get access to all of it. There is a strong sense of having to experience everything that I have always passed up in favor of safety and predictability. But some of those behaviors are not safe and not appropriate. I seem to be having the most trouble with the deep sense of what I have lost and was deprived of. Trouble accepting that it is just gone. Because I am not sure it is. It has recently become a raging battle.

I have spent a lot of time looking back on times gone by and trying to put the puzzle pieces together for myself. When this is the most intense, it is like having a videotape of my entire life being played in my head on fast forward. I have a photograph of me in my white high school graduation dress next to a dozen red roses in our living room in Virginia. I recently found it and spent some time examining it carefully. One evening, while looking at myself in the mirror, I had a vision of the moment of that photograph and my face actually transformed back to that barely sixteen-year-old girl in the mirror in front of my eyes. It didn't really scare me but seemed to connect my current self with that girl for the first time.

I even wrote to Michael at the hair salon when I was having my annual permanent.

I remain terrified that the perm will burn up my hair but so far that has never happened. I don't think there is a Trish without my long hair, do you?

How prophetic those words were.

As for my other problems, I am putting myself in professional hands today in an effort to deal with my strong feelings, tendencies, impulses, etc. I remember when Andrew was young, five or six, he always struggled to conform his enormous energy into a tolerable level for others. He came home from school one day with a carefully written paper that said "It's hard to be good, but I can do it." I feel just like that. I think I can but it's hard. There are all these things going on inside of me, feelings that belong to me alone, that I need to claim and to exercise. I have tried so many types of activities to satisfy those feelings but unsuccessfully. There is a capacity for certain things that can't find shape or form so they keep floating around inside, relentlessly controlling my inner emotional life. I know I should get them under control but, to be honest, I don't know if I want to. At least I'm not convinced yet. Sometimes it just feels good to be less than perfect, somewhat pathetic, needy, involved, caring and slightly out of control. I love the out of control part, having had so little experience with that in the past. But I still quickly make the proper adjustments to regain that control. In fact, you are probably noticing that in this very letter. How is that for honesty? Is your face contorted with confusion right now? Well if it is, too bad. I am sure you get it all anyway. Heck, I can't even think something without you figuring it out. Stop that. No, don't. God, I'm a wreck. Perhaps I can get cured in one hour at 3 pm today.

Michael wrote back to me:

Something has happened over the last few months. Your spiritual presence has been with me all along but I have begun to feel your physical self as well sometimes. Once it felt like you were at my side while walking along the street. It startled me the first time and I wasn't sure if it was just my imagination or that I was thinking of you at the time. But when it would happen with my mind on other things then I knew that you had the ability to be there. Wish I could transport myself that way. Can you hear me in your head at times during the day? I tend to have long conversations with you at different times. Sometimes I use it as a stress reliever. At the end of the day when heading home or to get a beer, I settle down to my chats with you. Thankfully they don't take place out loud.

Summer arrived and I couldn't wait to get to the shore.

Dear Michael,

I am, thank God, on the plane heading for San Diego. Last week was indescribably difficult. Words just can't say. I feel as bad physically as I can ever remember without actually being sick. The enormous stress of work has exhausted me in a scary kind of way. I tried to keep it under control and did for a while but then it just got away from me. Impossible to sleep, don't feel like eating, so what started as a little diet to make sure I'd look good on the beach turned into a real weight loss which even I know has gone far enough. Mark gently suggests that I have a slight tendency towards anorexia, especially when under so much stress. He's probably right in that I feel somehow empowered by not eating.

On Thursday I briefly lost my ability to be good as you instructed and I have been paying for it in a big way ever since. The amazing thing was that I had a few days to contemplate my actions before Thursday and the night before, you appeared to me in a very vivid dream. You didn't walk into the room, instead you kind of floated in slow motion while all the others of us walked normally. You were surrounded by a warm but strong light. I didn't seem to be expecting you but when I saw you, I was filled with joy. I know that this dream was your way of trying to protect me and help me believe in the goodness of me, but I'm a tough case, you know. I should never have added Thursday's behavior to an already deeply vulnerable state of mind. But there were some dramatic and hopefully permanent lessons learned.

In some ways, I think I've had a bit of a mini-nervous breakdown. Instead of being hospitalized, and I've prayed for that, I am going to God's natural hospital, my beautiful place on the shore. It is there and only there that I feel I can recover and rediscover myself. I'm still floating emotionally, trying to recover from all the trauma before I left, trying to get back on track. Sometimes I wonder if I can ever walk back into that office again. That life can be so barren that I fit into it things that attempt to connect me with someone or something. Needless to say, the wrong things and the wrong people sometimes.

Today I feel as though I have risen above my own life and myself and am looking down on it. Almost like being dead in a way, I imagine. Now I desperately want to wake up.

Michael began to write more openly to me:

You don't sound too convinced of my ability to listen and talk with you about your needs and desires. I'm not sure how to give you that peace of mind but eventually I will find the key and you will open the floodgates and find a release. You think that I am holding back, maybe some, but I am very open to you. More so than I have been with anyone. You need a lift in your emotions, I need to give it to you. I don't go anywhere without you with me. Visually you are etched into my memories. You have always had my love and will continue to have it. It is richer for me now than at any other time.

I kept the dialogue going:

I love the way you are beginning to share more with me and in some ways I am amazed by what is under those layers. When I said I was afraid, I meant it. I believe I know where this is headed more clearly than you. It seems that, in slightly different ways, we are both waking up at the same time. And we are each being gently and lovingly nudged awake by the other. The problem is that once you wake up, your needs change dramatically and it is much more difficult to manage. So while I have been resisting exactly what I'm feeling now, I'm starting to lose my ability to do so. And I want to open the door wide between us, but I have deep concerns. For both of us, but especially you. I will be better able to adjust to the new feelings than you. Perhaps the best thing to do is buy some art supplies. You may be moving into a very creative period!

Up until fairly recently, it was simply impossible to allow anyone inside me due to the ongoing threat to everything female about me followed by my "transformation" only to discover that my life did not accommodate what is very much the essence of me. I feel myself slipping towards you more, and every instinct I have tells me to slow down and back off, but I'm having trouble. We will both get hurt, maybe not by each other, but by the situation itself. Do you know this? It already hurts, doesn't it?

Love,

(I don't know how to sign at this moment)

In response, Michael wrote:

This past 6-10 months have allowed me to clarify many aspects of my life, past and present. Even though you aren't quite sure whether to believe it, I've always had you as part of my psyche and in my thoughts. This past year with us talking and confiding and me being able to open up without fear of being misread or misunderstood has been wonderful. I have missed the emotional and psychic relationship that I had always felt with you. It was something I yearned for and was afraid that one misstep would break the thread that I always held onto.

My Vietnam project, now a film, was shown on PBS and had attracted the attention of Andrew Lloyd Weber's Really Useful Company in New York City. They asked me to come to the city in the fall to discuss the project with them. I was unbelievably thrilled and Michael had agreed to take the train up with me from Baltimore where I would attend a professional conference first.

Dear Michael,

Mark and I went to our favorite Spanish restaurant, Such is Life, last night. I get so much attention from the owners and our waiter. He already knows everything I like to eat and drink without my having to order. I get countless hugs and kisses, upon arrival, upon departure and sometimes in between. They send a long stemmed rose home with me which I always put by my bed to wake up to the next morning. There are wonderful classical Spanish guitarists and sometimes a flute as well. It is always a lovely experience but I often get depressed afterwards. The Latin men who own and run the restaurant are so unbelievably passionate and affectionate, just like James, and I just want to absorb all of that completely and constantly. Mark kind of sits back and watches all of this, enjoying the way they treat me, but like he is an outsider, isolated somehow. And when we have to leave, I feel like the outsider, isolated from all of them when I really want to be part of them. And, in my heart, I believe I am part of them in a way. I just can't break out. It is very difficult for me not to be acting on these feelings. Very difficult. I am very tired of saying no, no to everything I am feeling inside.

Anyway, my current vow is to stay very busy, get a lot of things done, and prepare for my trip in October. I, too, am counting the days, so looking forward to it. This time next month, it will be time. I am estimating the time in many different ways. Weeks and weekends, cycles, goals to be accomplished by then, etc. Exactly five weeks from right now, we will already be settled in New York, hopefully out in the city, not cold, maybe sitting in some pub, talking, or maybe not even talking. Just happy.

Dear Trish,

We've been talking to each other more lately. Your self is coming through more often and I am beginning to sense the duality that drives you, and concerns you. I say that I sense it but that doesn't mean I have knowledge of what exactly this duality consists of. I feel a strong alliance between us and am grateful that you've let me into some regions that you are sensitive with. My understanding of your resolve to not be put in a place of pain or hurt is real.

Because you push forward and then pull back before the next need arises, it is as if I'm riding a swell, not a wave. It is the lull in between that allows me time to diagnose your needs and try to decipher the mystery within your sometimes cryptic clues. I suppose that is what a clue is meant to be, cryptic. If it wasn't, it would be an answer. Something we are both searching for.

You deserve so much for what you have endured and managed to hold together. At some point the weight has to be shifted somewhere other than on your shoulders. Survival is a need to soar without guilt. Go away to whatever place or space in life's drama that is needed. No, demanded, because without it you will die little bits at a time inside.

That is what concerns me about the situation within you. I'm afraid of the little cracks becoming fractures. I don't know yet if any of us close to you have the alchemy to mix the ointment in order to heal the cracks before they widen.

Michael had no idea how intuitive he really was. My cracks were about to widen beyond my wildest imagination.

EVERYTHING AFTER

When I live at the shore, where life makes perfect sense, I get used to the constant sound of the ocean, coming in and going out, waves breaking. At certain moments, when I am conscious of it, it can actually be annoying and I long for quiet. Then there is that slight pause, a hesitation, which creates a sudden and surprising silence. The very moment I was diagnosed with cancer was like a version of that silence that lasted for months. In the noisy ebb and flow of my troubled existence, that quiet was the break that I needed and longed for. The silence, the bubble created by my disease, in which I could exist, protecting me until I could learn to take care of myself.

CHAPTER FIFTY-ONE

In my letter to Michael, I write about how I lost my ability to be good on a Thursday. And how I had a few days to contemplate it beforehand. It was almost the only thing I could think of. I go to my therapist who is now fully up to speed on the "duality" of my life, and state bluntly that I am going to see James on Thursday and this time I am going to go through with it, to put myself, and him, out of our misery. I begin to cry from the sheer agony of my declaration. He first gives me a box of Kleenex, and then becomes angry with me, demanding to know why I would ever consciously choose to be so self-destructive. He flatly tells me that this decision will ruin my life, make me a permanent victim to my abuse and to my father's influence. He reminds me of my wonderful life, my devoted family who adores me, and my potential for happiness. But I cannot hear it, although I am there with the vague hope that perhaps he can find a way to reach me when I have not been able to reach myself. He can't.

I arrive in the dreary, cheap motel room where James is waiting. He takes off all his clothes but I do not. He does handle me gently, assuming I will finally succumb. But when he shows himself to me, there is no way I can take him inside me and accept his issue. I dig as deeply inside myself as I possibly can and refuse to proceed. Aroused by his anticipation and fueled by his disappointment, he brings himself to an orgasm in his cupped hand while I retreat to the dresser, putting my hand up my skirt to finish alone. There is absolutely no connection between us, which is what makes it easier and what makes it so devastating. He washes his hands and dresses. He is not kind.

I stand still in the middle of the room while my life, my essence drops through the tips of my toes, like a robe slipping from my shoulders, completely emptying me inside. It is at this moment that I invite cancer in to visit. I instantly begin to create my tumor, the mass that will encompass all my pain and suffering and abuse and lust and self-loathing. It is as if all of these emotions begin a rush to my breast. I have somehow managed to save myself in that dreary room by finally rejecting my own version of my father's daughter, by rejecting James who may as well be my father by this time. My knees are so watery that it is difficult to put my shoes on and actually walk out the door.

CHAPTER FIFTY-TWO

Within three days, the tumor I made in my final appearance at a dumpy motel room trying to live up to my birthright, appears in my right breast. It isn't subtle. There are knots and lumps and my breast is hot and swollen. Mark looks at it and it is clear that he knows that I have finally done it.

My right breast, covered with the port wine stain has always been temperamental, an exaggerated version of whatever is going on in my female life. When it produced milk for my two sons, it was burning hot and brick hard. It was always more tender than the other more well behaved breast at that time of the month, lumpier and heavier. It has always had a life of its own.

I go to my gynecologist, who has seen my right breast misbehave plenty of times in the past. He says it is engorged and cystic, let's watch it for thirty days and then come back. So I watch my cancer thrive unattended and buy the next bra size to accommodate its rapid growth. When I come back, exactly thirty days later, the doctor opens the gown, takes one look at my tumor, closes it, backs up from the examining table, and says it is time to see the surgeon. Right now.

The surgeon closes the gown after a brief exam and retreats backwards all the way to the far corner of the room to "chat." How odd that my tumor seems to make doctors walk backwards. He says I need a biopsy, not next week, but right away.

I am sent next door to have an ultrasound. The tech places the paddle on my breast, looks up at the monitor, turns ghostly pale, and immediately excuses herself. She returns with a very nervous smile and says I am free to go. Dead giveaway.

The biopsy is scheduled for Friday and it is hard to wait. By this time, my tumor is so pervasive even at its young age that it can be easily spotted through my clothing, almost twice the size of the other. I spend evenings with a bag of frozen peas on it to reduce the swelling and discomfort. It is on fire.

Waiting for my biopsy to begin, a wonderful nurse tells me she has been through the same thing and not to worry. Most aren't cancer. I cling to that, knowing full well it is completely untrue in my case. I speak with a member of the surgical team to let him know that I do not wish to be sedated (never in a room full of men I don't know) and want to go only with the local anesthetic. He seems skeptical but does not refuse. After being wheeled into a small, cold operating room, my face is covered with a heavy blue surgical sheet. I can hear the surgeon enter the room, but no one tells him that I am wide awake and fully conscious under my blue sheet. So he speaks freely to the others, noting how much the incision is bleeding, possibly due to my birthmark, which he seems to find fascinating. The plan is to remove a piece of the tumor and send it to the lab, with results expected back within twenty-four hours. But when he sees my tumor, he orders a frozen section, opting to wait for an immediate result. I hear him chatting with the others, waiting for the phone to ring. The call comes in. He returns to the table, saying nothing. Nothing. I realize that he doesn't know that I am wide awake. So I ask, *is it benign?* He says simply, no, shocked to hear my voice coming from under the blue sheet.

What happens to me at that moment is as clear to me today as it was in that cold operating room years ago. At first it is overwhelming relief, spontaneous and consuming. I feel a very powerful, spiritual presence fold me in its aura, giving me an immediate sense of peace. And faith, a very real thing, presents itself, filling me with the belief that I will get sick to get well. Completely well from the sickness of my life. And no matter how scary it is, or will get, not to worry. It will not take my life. I will be healed. And I choose to believe. This will be my story.

CHAPTER FIFTY-THREE

I do nothing but shake like a leaf for days after I am told the news. Can't eat a thing, can't sleep, can't stop shaking. Every moment that I am awake, which is every moment in the beginning, is torture because there is no way to process what I have been told, what we have been told. I long to be unconscious, run over by a truck, be transported to a tropical island, to be anywhere but in this life at this moment.

We lie in bed for the whole night, only dozing, hanging onto each other for dear life. I have always wanted this kind of closeness with my husband and he has never been able to give it. But now it is the most natural thing in the world. It is the first obvious blessing of cancer.

The following day I go to my office to inform my top three people, gradually realizing it as a mistake because how can I explain something I haven't even begun to process myself. The two women suggest that I tell the entire company openly right away. I am not at all sure about that, feeling a need for privacy. One of them cries quietly, the other in shock. I can see the now familiar "Thank God it isn't me" look on their faces. When I argue for privacy, one of them says, "Well, what are you going to do when your appearance starts to change?" First of many insensitive remarks that will be made along the way.

I take a call from my good friend in Hawaii, the one whom

I allowed to read my manuscript. He immediately asks what is wrong, hearing it in my voice. I say that it is bad, very bad. He asks if I want to talk about it. I say not now. He describes himself sitting with his partner on a terrace overlooking the ocean about to play a round of golf. I can feel the joy and peace in his voice and I can see the ocean in my wrecked mind. I offer some advice. Taste, feel, and appreciate every moment of that beautiful day he is having. Somehow he understands. I hang up so full of envy that I can hardly breathe. I know that I will never be that carefree, that peaceful, that happy again. My life is gone. I become so overwrought that I have to leave. I wonder if he still thinks my husband is a lucky man.

We go to the surgeon's office to hear confirmation of the pathology report. It is Friday afternoon. He is winding down for the week and his office is empty except for us. His nurse is not gracious. I get the feeling maybe they have stayed open only to see me and my powerful tumor. He comes in after keeping us waiting for a while with my file folder in his hand and a yellow "stickie" on it with the name of a type of carcinoma or something. I guess that is my pathology report. It doesn't bear my name and he never opens the folder to look at any report. He draws a picture of a breast on the front cover of the file folder showing my type of cancer in the ducts. If it is confined to the ducts, he says, it is one hundred percent curable, no problem. But that is not the kind I have. (So why tell me about that one first?) No, mine has invaded the walls (what walls?), and that reduces my chances down to fifty percent. We look so shocked that he shrugs his shoulder and says, okay, sixty percent. (Well, which is it?) He also mentions possible spread to who knows how many places in my body and he casually names them, like lungs, lymph nodes, bones, etc. He does repeat, however, that my lymph nodes feel "real normal" and it very well may be confined to the breast. (Yeah, I feel a lot better now.) He also mentions that the tumor is about two months old. (I already know that.) He proceeds by saying that the tumor is way too large to remove surgically right now, that it would be just too "messy." He is thinking that we treat it with chemotherapy for a few months and see if it will shrink up "real nice" and then remove it later. (Leave that hot, raging, huge tumor inside of me after I went to so much trouble to get rid of everything that is inside of it? How fast can we get out of here?)

He refers us to the "good ole boy" network oncologist who treated three friends of mine in the past two years. They are all dead. We object. He mentions the option of the Mayo Clinic. It is the first thing that feels right about this hideous meeting. I ask for an immediate referral.

CHAPTER FIFTY-FOUR

I am devastated after that appointment, still overwhelmed by the possibility, in my mind the probability, of death. Live with that for a few days and it becomes easier to adjust to the side effects of chemotherapy. One of my first angels, Glynnis, calls out of the blue and talks to Mark. She is a surgical recovery nurse, has heard of my diagnosis, and wonders if she might help. She is an eleven year survivor of breast cancer herself. She leaves her number. Mark and I are lying on the bed and as he is telling me this, he bursts into tears. He sobs and then apologizes. I am relieved and it gives me comfort to comfort him. He takes off to the store and I am left in my room alone.

I get a message from Heidi, another angel, from the Mayo Clinic. I call her immediately. She has a warm, supportive way about her and says we can be seen at the Breast Clinic on Wednesday by a radiation oncologist who is a woman, and she adds, a very neat lady. I am so relieved by talking with Heidi not only because I figure we will be among friends there, but I long at this point to discuss treatment with a woman. She mentions that the Clinic would like to have forty-eight hours to see all of my films and my actual pathology slides, not just the yellow stickie. I am overjoyed to be out of the good ole boy network and in a more elite place where I feel I will be better understood. I immediately begin making arrangements to have the slides sent over from the local lab. It is difficult and I have to become very assertive when the clerk tells me that if they are going to go somewhere else, a pathologist has to review them. I ask if a pathologist hasn't already reviewed them or how would we have a report? She nervously says that he has to "re-review" them. I hang up the phone and feel more like myself than I have in days, very empowered by making my own arrangements.

By evening, Mark and I are totally exhausted, depressed, in shock, and closer than we have ever been before. Bonded completely. I feel like I am living inside of him, drawing off his strength and health, being beautifully protected. I am almost afraid to be away from him, not because I feel dependent, but because I believe without him I might disappear into nothing. We decide that we will try to eat something as both boys are out for the evening, and then we will go to our bed to watch the 20/20 interview with Christopher Reeve who has had a riding accident leaving him paralyzed from the neck down. We assume this will make us feel very lucky. Then we have a Valium ritual together. I take half of five milligrams, and he takes a whole. We fall asleep peacefully, me in a matter of moments. I wake up about four hours later, shaking all over, and he gently insists that I take the other half. It takes a little longer than the first time, but I sleep for four more glorious hours.

The rest allows me to wake Saturday morning feeling more positive and energetic even though I have many physical ailments. I talk to a close friend, a Vietnam combat vet, who has been battling serious illness for some time. He is so wise and comforting that our talk feels like a brief trip to heaven and back. He says not to confuse the "c" word with the "d" word.

Peter and I go to Ted's Hot Dogs for lunch just like we do every Saturday. I want him to feel as normal as possible. He orders for me for the first time because he knows what I always get. A small gesture of protectiveness that I find very touching.

We carefully stage the scene for when my mother will arrive to pick up Pete for birthday shopping. I am out washing the car so she will not come in the house and stay too long. She comes up to me, teary eyed, talking non-stop about breast cancer there in the yard in front of my boys, me with the hose in my hand. We are all smiling at the predictability of her response and she hands over two books she has brought along. After they leave, I go inside and look up what I believe to be my case in one of the books, a very technical medical manual of some sort. My survival percentage comes in at forty-one percent. I begin to shake again, violently this time, and gag and cry. When I go to the gym, where Mark is already working out, I can't ride the bike because my chest is too tight and I feel like throwing up. He looks so concerned. I just give up and go home, trying not to crash further.

I make dinner reservations for us in our usual place, thinking it will be fun for us to get out. Mark is skeptical but I am insistent, saying it is my treat to him. I dress up to look pretty, defiantly wearing a tight, striped shirt. Hair long and loose. We get our usual affectionate attention from the owner and his staff. I run into a client who originally recommended the place to us. We chat and he says I look good. He repeatedly asks about my father and his health. Oh, the irony.

It is wonderful for us to be out for that dinner. We are close, heads together, savoring every moment of the delicious food, Spanish music, good friends. When we return home, Peter comes in from his evening with friends and lays with us in our bed to tell all about it. He has done that at least a hundred times before but what has always seemed like such a small moment suddenly becomes very profound. He is conflicted inside, I know, because it will be his sixteenth birthday in a few days and he is so excited. And now cancer has intruded on that. He wants to be sensitive but I know he feels cheated. I vow to make sure his birthday is fun and normal.

Sunday I crash hard, have a very bad day. We try to go to a movie at the neighborhood theatre but a woman dies shortly into the film and the funeral scene is too devastating for me to watch. I have to leave my seat. I cannot appropriately recover so I insist on walking home. Mark looks stunned and unsure about whether he should leave with me. I say no, he should stay for the rest of the film.

I cry quietly to myself on the walk home but crave the physical activity. I cannot get myself together and pause at the bridge overlooking the lake, the exact same place where I stood under the moon the first night that I let James kiss me. I decide to call a close friend, my nutritionist, to express my fears that my tight chest is really lung cancer, and that my lower back ache is not really from shaking for three days straight feeling tense as a board, but instead is a tumor growing on my spine. He assures me that these feelings are normal and also absolutely untrue. It is a depressed immune system in great shock allowing bad fall allergies to wreak havoc. He promises me that between nutrition, chemotherapy, and my amazing strength and attitude, we can and will overcome this together. I feel so much better that my physical symptoms lessen.

I go to the dance studio and am relieved to find that my body still works beautifully, the music runs through me, and the smell of the wood floor intoxicates me. The workout makes my breast feel hot and flushed, but I feel wonderful. My senses have never been so full of life.

CHAPTER FIFTY-FIVE

Glynnis, the angel, comes over with a tasteful and helpful video about survivors and their chemotherapy experience. She is a robust redhead, with lots of wavy hair, and a ton of spunk. I like her immediately. She had a large tumor also that had spread into her lymph nodes which she diagnosed herself in a dream. During a routine chest x-ray, they also found lung cancer. She is well now. She is reassuring. She tells me several times I will be okay. I believe her.

We buy thousands of vitamins and I start my pre-chemo regimen to make me a wonder of medical science, which is my intention. Boy, this is a full time job. Mark is tired so I clean up the kitchen. We grocery shop together, share everything. He is talking more than in the last twenty years combined. I have always wanted this with him. It is so pleasurable.

CHAPTER FIFTY-SIX

Mark keeps the appointment with the good ole boy local killer oncologist. He returns to me (I wouldn't go), ashen with no lips. He said if my tumor came from somewhere else to my breast, I have a ten percent chance of survival. My gynecologist says that tumors originate in the breast. (Shouldn't the good ole boy know that?)

I speak to a lesbian doctor, very tough, at a major university medical facility who says her plan would be massive doses of chemotherapy. As much as I can tolerate without actually killing me. It doesn't seem to fit into my healing story. I don't think so.

We go to the Mayo Clinic and meet Lana, a lovely nurse, and the doctor who is a radiation oncologist. Speaking quietly, she says in a ridiculously calm tone with a little reassuring smile that I have an eleven centimeter tumor, grade something (too high), and we should consider immediate surgery. She intuitively sees the distance between us and knows I need something else, someone else. She excuses herself and drags in Dr. John. He's the one. I know right away. He takes my case. (I would later find out that he is her husband. Sensing that he was a perfect match for me, she found him in the hall, asked him to come in, and he refused. They argued vehemently. He was not taking new patients and did not want to meet me. Thank God she prevailed.)

We go to the Mayo surgeon next. It's Wednesday. How's Friday for us, he asks. I negotiate to be allowed to go to New York in two weeks as planned to meet with Andrew Lloyd Weber's company. He says I will have to earn it. I promise that I will.

I refuse a request for a medical photograph of my raging right breast. I am very shaky.

My friend, Vicky, the woman who had worked for me with whom I shared a sexual abuse history, says that my tumor is my own abuse taking shape and form. She says I will leave it on the altar of the operating table and I will wake up free. She says I will get exactly the right amount of cancer that I need to be healed. Faith appears again. Vicky is another of my angels, tainted but powerful.

Friday I'm ready. No fear, no depression. Surgery is delayed so I wear two gowns to ensure ass coverage and alternate between ballet and stand up comedy in the waiting room. My parents laugh through their fear.

I beg for Mark to be allowed to accompany me to pre-op. They agree. I disappear with the help of the drugs.

When I awake, my boys are in my room. They laugh at how confused I am, in and out.

My mother stays with me in my room all night. I'm grateful. She reminds me of the mom she used to be before I uncovered the family secret. I awake early. She is asleep in the recliner covered by a thin blanket. The sun is shining through the window on her.

I wait for the realization that it is gone, my breast. But I like it, I feel light. Dr. John visits me and says indications are at least one bad node. We'll know more in a few days.

Mark takes me home and takes care of me. Bathes me. We're not upset by what we see. He washes my long hair in the tub.

We are waiting to hear. Mom and I walk in on Mark who is leaning on the kitchen counter with the phone to his ear. Head in hand. "Oh, no!" he says. I say quietly under my breath, "I'm dead." Eighteen infected lymph nodes of the forty that were removed. Huge tumor. My mother is stunned. She leaves us alone. I cry. We are terrified. But Doctor John says that a bone marrow transplant may offer "significant hope." Oh, God.

My drains come out faster than the surgeon has ever seen. No fluid to be aspirated after that. He says I can travel if I can touch my ear with that arm. I do. It hurts like hell. I'm going to New York!

CHAPTER FIFTY-SEVEN

Cancer will not be allowed to take my long planned trip to Baltimore and New York away from me. One of my main concerns is that I have already bought some new clothes for the trip and am not sure how my new one-breasted status will work with my typical tight body suits. I am thrilled to discover that the prosthesis looks so natural that I will be able to wear any of my clothes and feel comfortable. Mark takes me to the airport and I am not the least bit sure that I can possibly leave him behind at a time like this. But the meeting in New York is the future. I have to move in that direction. I can't give an inch to cancer.

My diagnosis shakes Michael to his core and he is finding it very difficult to cope. While driving home in a bad rainstorm, he pulls over to the side of the road, breaks down in tears, and weeps. He is keeping a journal of his own for me, in a beautiful small notebook with thick grey lined pages, in his own hand. On the cover is his original artwork, painted in grey and lavender with a hint of turquoise on the front, and pink with dark grey on the back. Ironically he starts the journal just a few short weeks before my diagnosis, and in his writing is a strong premonition. He continues to write after he finds out.

There are instances, as you suspect, when I know what you are thinking. I can sense your feelings. There is a clarity with some emotions and it can't be explained. Acknowledging only makes it seem a parlor trick or someone trying to be sensitive. I do know. I know before we talk.

You have taught me to allow some moments to take place spontaneously. This way they become magic which then becomes art. That point, that moment, is exactly what I am searching for. This connection is glued by some substance other than something feral. As much as I want the physical, it is the mystical that magically moves me.

You are in the air and so is anticipation. You are on your way to Baltimore and I am looking forward to seeing you Sunday. The last we spoke you showed concern about this trip and how I will react to everything. You continue to voice fears that I haven't any idea what I am about to experience and/or see. Maybe even to feel. You are right and I will grant you that concern. There is no way I can possibly know what it will be like. I am coming to you with an open mind. I may not be prepared because you can't tell me how to be or for what. To me it doesn't matter. It is obvious in how you voice concern that it does matter very much to you.

New York is a fitting place for us to spend this time together. It is a neutral place we both love and appreciate for the energy it has. Besides, it is a place that I have wonderful memories of the two of us spending time together getting to know each other better, listening and talking and you working me over to get me to open up. Your frustration level must have been high after that trip. This one won't have any frustration or stress.

My first stop is Baltimore for a professional conference. I have confided what I am going through to a male friend from Australia whom I had met at a prior conference. He has a serious crush on me and seems to have high expectations about what will take place during this conference rendezvous. (What he doesn't know is how very easy it will be to say no to all that after my experience of repeatedly rejecting James.) A successful, wealthy, sophisticated man, he greets me warmly and arranges for a quiet dinner for us at a small restaurant. I speak openly about what is happening to me and how it is changing my view of the world. He shares emotional stories of his own father. He watches over me, holds my arm when we are walking on the street, careful to make sure he isn't hurting me. We don't talk much; he is just there for me.

He invites me out with another couple who knows nothing of my situation and I endure a terrible evening of listening to the three of them plan their fabulous vacations and future endeavors. All I can think of is that I may never have another vacation and planning for the future seems an uncertain luxury at best. When we return to the hotel, I cry and try to express my fears to my friend but I can tell that his patience is wearing thin and this is not the conference he has fantasized about. How is he to know that his fantasy was never going to become reality anyway? I am certain I probably led him on, but who cares now?

My emotional state deteriorates and I make sudden plans to take the Amtrak to DC for a few hours to see Michael. I cannot wait the extra days for our first planned meeting. Even though my train arrives early and he is not sure which one I am on, he is right there when I arrive and his face is a welcome sight. His hug tells me that he will give me every ounce of strength, love and energy he can muster. He offers plenty of emotional space, but always keeps a close eye in case I am tired, hungry, cold, uncomfortable or in need of anything at all. He is like medicine to me.

After my conference concludes, we take the train to New York, saying very little. He has found a wonderful hotel across the street from the Empire State Building, completely remodeled in an art deco theme. We have a spacious suite with two bedrooms. Mark is okay with it because he trusts me and wants me to have someone close by. Michael lets me choose the big open bedroom with the two beds next to the huge picture windows overlooking the street. Beginning to realize that I have probably taken on too much by traveling so soon after my surgery, I am exhausted and in some discomfort. It is a beautiful, sunny, cool autumn day and I immediately open the windows and sit at the foot of the bed, letting the cool breeze in. I lay back, eyes closed and I feel his hands begin to gently brush my face and stroke my hair. It makes me cry because I feel so much pain and fear, because my body is so torn apart, and because I trust him so completely. His feelings for me are pure and clean and decent, matching the new feeling I have in my own body since I rid myself of the abuse filled tumor. He takes a lot of time caressing me with his fingertips, giving both comfort and pleasure.

I am feeling uncomfortable in my travel clothes with the prosthesis rubbing against my raw surgical area so I change into my baggy pajamas. This allows Michael to place his hands on my bare skin, gently brushing my back and tracing the line of my new scar with deep care. His hands are intuitive and know exactly how and where the touch heals. It is intimate and beyond sexual, having none of the same meaning I am used to. We sleep in our own rooms at night but I know when I get up to go into the bathroom that he is awake and aware of exactly where I am and what I am doing. I know he checks on me when I am sleeping, and stops to watch my breath move in and out. His presence casts a protective spell on me. There is absolutely no doubt that I will accept this gift from him and it is absolutely necessary for him to give it. I sometimes feel that my spirit leaves my tired, beleaguered body and soars under the care of his sensitive, artistic and loving hands. It makes me feel like one of the thousands of pieces of fine art that he has handled in his career, like he is molding and shaping me to wellness, wholeness and joy. There is a rightness about it that I have waited my entire life to experience.

Only once does his hand reach to a sexual part of me and with his quiet searching and body "listening," he brings me to a long, slow climax that leaves me sobbing with complex emotions. I quickly call my husband to tell him that I have just experienced a celestial healing. What I tell him is true and he knows it without asking me to explain. A single orgasm that is not linked to sex, lust, desire or marriage cleanses me of the feeling that I am either a sexual being or a failure as a sexual being. He gives me the gift of joyful realization of pure sexual self without a hint of anything bad. He asks for nothing in return. I begin to feel the inside of my body brightening up, flowing more freely, returning to its original state. It is breathtaking. It is pure love.

CHAPTER FIFTY-EIGHT

I get dressed and prepare for my meeting with The Really Useful Company about my Vietnam project, the reason for my trip. Michael helps me hail a cab, preferring that I not deal with the New York subway in my condition. I do not mention my recent diagnosis in the meeting and for a brief time, forget that I have cancer in favor of pitching my beloved project as an artist. I feel exactly like myself and they are enthusiastic. I rush back to the hotel, excited to tell Michael all about it. He is waiting in the room, seated by the window at the small table in the waning light of day, dressed in shirt and tie for our planned evening out. He is smiling, as if he already knows that it has gone well. He takes great pleasure in my detailed recollection of the meeting.

I change into my little black dress, throw on my favorite leather jacket over it, and we head to the famous Rainbow and Stars cabaret at the top of the RCA building to celebrate. The view is spectacular and the entertainment is Amanda McBroom, singing with piano. I have a filet, perfectly cooked, and eat to my heart's content. Michael has a fruit and cheese plate and shares with me.

Not realizing that Amanda is a songwriter as well as a highly regarded cabaret singer, I am surprised to discover that she wrote "The Rose" theme song for the film of the same name. Her performance of the song is tender and moving and touches me deeply.

Some say love, it is a river that drowns the tender reed,
Some say love, it is a razor, that leaves your soul to bleed
Some say love, it is a hunger, an endless aching need
I say love, it is a flower, and you, its only seed

It's the heart afraid of breaking, that never learns to dance
It's the dream afraid of waking, that never takes the chance
It's the one who won't be taken,
  the one who can't seem to give
And the soul afraid of dying, that never learns to live

When the night has been too lonely,
  and the road has been too long
And you think that love is only for the lucky and the strong
Just remember in the winter, far beneath the bitter snow
Lies the seed that with the sun's love,
  in the spring becomes the rose

The experience is so pleasurable, so joyful, that I can barely breathe. We are very happy in a way that can only happen when you fully realize how very precious a moment is.

We return to Washington on the train and I prepare to fly back home. I am facing an unpleasant bone marrow biopsy early the next morning to determine whether the cancer has spread and whether I will be able to be my own donor for the transplant. It is necessary for me to go through the exercise of saying that I may decide to fly to Europe instead of home to the West because I might choose to decline all of the aggressive treatment planned for me and just go on an extended holiday instead. It is a game I play with myself to prove that I have a choice. Michael plays along but knows that I am going home to face my disease and all it symbolizes. Even so, I think he is relieved when I board the plane headed to Phoenix, back to my family. The parting is deeply painful and I leave a piece of myself there with him.

CHAPTER FIFTY-NINE

Mark rubs the back of my legs while the nurse digs around inside my bone, trying to capture a little piece of it along with a sample of the marrow using an instrument that looks like an egg beater. The first time she hooks a piece, she drops it on the way out and has to start over. The area outside the bone can be anesthetized but there is no way to deaden the inside. It is a dull, aching pain. I don't need a biopsy to tell me that my bone marrow is clean, healthy, kicking and beautiful which I can easily see when she shows me the small tube full of the gorgeous life that just came out of me.

Dr. John cautiously explains Mayo's recommended protocol of a "stem cell rescue," a type of bone marrow transplant. There are still a few tests left to rule out the presence of cancer in any other part of my body besides the tumor and surrounding lymph nodes, which is a requirement to qualify for the treatment, but so far everything seems to suggest that I am the perfect candidate. I easily meet the standard of at least ten infected nodes with my impressive eighteen.

I listen carefully to how it works. It is assumed that my immune system has been compromised by the cancer in the nodes being circulated throughout my body by way of the lymph system. Those cancer cells can be hiding anywhere. I will be subjected to high dose chemotherapy for four days non-stop to completely kill my immune system. Once my numbers bottom out after several days, I will then receive back into my body my own stem cells collected in advance from my clean, healthy bone marrow. Hopefully these stem cells will jump-start the making of a brand new immune system, which I will tend to in a sterile room. Healing myself, starting over, choosing just exactly what I may like to kill off along with my old immune system, and being completely responsible for recreating myself, rebirthing myself. I know before he is even finished speaking that this is my healing path. My transplant coordinator shakes her head and says that no one ever wants to go through a bone marrow transplant, that she is usually quite unpopular. But I am certain of it. In my heart I know that this is why I am sick, so that I may have this opportunity. That therein lies my physical and spiritual healing. The next chapter of my story.

CHAPTER SIXTY

But first things first. I will have two rounds of aggressive outpatient chemotherapy, three weeks apart, beginning on Halloween. I will have a short break the week before Christmas while I collect my stem cells. Then two more chemo treatments, followed as soon as possible by the transplant.

My journal continues to be a lifeline.

October 29th

After a major sinker in the mid-afternoon yesterday that lasted quite a while, I took off for the dance studio for a very good workout. I put on my favorite sweatshirt and pushed the arm further than before, working through the discomfort, grunting and groaning. My reward was the great benefit of progress, the arm feeling so much looser and more normal after. It is stiff this morning but I will go through the whole drill again today. I love the studio so much. It is a lifesaver for me. I am in a major pshyc-up mode for Tuesday morning's first chemo treatment and also for the dreaded doctor visit on Monday afternoon. I will find out if all my test results are clean so that we can plan for the stem cell rescue. I am trying to take fear out of it as much as possible. I will be ready by Tuesday morning with the proper attitude. I have always hated Halloween.

October 31st

I am terrified of allowing them to push the chemo drugs through my vein. I make them check and double-check the dosage. I don't even like to take aspirin. Mark rubs my feet and watches me closely when they place the IV needle and open the line. First it feels like I will faint and then just this full, sickening, overwhelming misery. I pee radioactive orange.

When I return home, Andrew and Peter are on the patio carving pumpkins.

November 5th

Despite how bad I feel right away, it is nothing compared to how I feel after the first twenty-four hours passes. The nausea is uncontrollable. For days, it is horrible. Truly horrible. I have to focus with all my power and continue to visualize chemo as my ally, not my enemy. I know that my nutrition is replacing the friendly fast-growing cells that are being killed along with the cancer cells. I also know that the misery is temporary. Chemo is my army of foot soldiers, coursing through my veins, obliterating the enemy. I join up with chemo and just try to hang on. It passes.

November 9th

Today I am so full of joy and life and love and hope that I am about to burst. As I got out of my beautiful car and walked the short distance to my office door, I threw my face to the brilliant blue desert autumn sky and soaked up the energy of the sun. The last few nights it has been the enormous and powerful energy of the full moon.

It is this life-altering event that has allowed me to grasp and feel and experience things each and every moment of each and every day. I love waking up in the morning, getting up in the night to go to the bathroom and then slipping back into bed to fall asleep, chatting about the most mundane teenage things with Peter which he does incessantly, trying to understand the fantastic creative complexities of Andrew, soaking up the enormous affection of the people who are not afraid to love me and whose love I am able to accept, having trivial conversations with my employees, feeling the power of healing I have within myself to remold and reshape my life free of all the pain and conflict of my past, listening to the Beatles full blast on my car stereo.

November 12ᵗʰ

I received a message from the Mayo Clinic late Friday afternoon saying that not only did the insurance company approve the transplant, but all my pre-transplant tests came back "perfect." What a relief. I could feel myself going from just hanging on with hope and prayer to turning with the tailwind and facing the cure and the future without so much anxiety. I know that the insurance company does not pay to prolong life. Only if they feel certain the procedure has the chance to cure.

I went shopping Saturday and in a dressing room, trying on a turtleneck, pulled out my first full handful of hair. It was terrifying and traumatic as hell, but I've been waiting for it and am now in the mode of let's get on with it so there is one less thing to dread. It continues to come out and now I have to deal with the logistics of the situation in the next few days. Scary stuff that requires bravery and courage of a new kind. My scalp feels so funny, like I am wearing my hair. Gotta let it go.

So I had a major cry, mourning the loss of my long hair, and then went to the studio and had a hard core talk with my disease. I explained in a loud, stern voice to cancer that I was willing to give up my breast and go ahead and take my hair but that's it. The rest is mine and I am not giving anything else. In fact, just as a statement, I am taking my hair before cancer gets a chance. I will never be a victim again.

November 15ᵗʰ

My head is completely off focus right now and I am feeling a strong urge to write like crazy to help find my way through this. Perhaps it is the low white cell count blues. Gosh, my red cells are decent so between good red, low white, and the plain old blues, we have the American flag.

Mark just called me to breakfast (fried egg, two pancakes, orange juice, antibiotic, and 14 vitamins). Peter was doing his homework at the table complaining about not caring about the evolution of Japanese and European feudalism or some such thing which I agreed was not particularly relevant to me or my life unless it had to do with white blood cells, at which point he wanted to know why I didn't care about black blood cells or was I prejudiced or something and the whole thing kind of deliciously deteriorated from that point on.

I gave Mayo a call to ask the questions that have been bothering me. The nurse said the low white count could be lower and it was very good that the platelets and red cells were not low because that would allow the white cells to bounce back faster. She said I could do things as I felt like it and although the low count could make me more tired, staying in bed and cutting everything back would not necessarily make the count rise. So I am going to a deep stretch dance class this morning. If it doesn't feel good, I will leave, or if anyone has a cold or something like that.

My hair dresser and I held hands, cried, and she took the scissors to my very long hair which was falling out in clumps in her hand. I am very proud that I was able to go through with the loss of my long hair, which was a huge letting go step for me, very cleansing and healing. The soft waves that were underneath were such a surprise, like a reward and make me feel special.

I woke up at 2 am just flipped out over my white cells. Imagining the worst, I got the shakes and couldn't get it back together. Mark made every attempt to help, but isn't sure sometimes. When I would have preferred a gentle back rub and lots of quiet "everything is going to be okay" with no logic and no medical speculation, he instead suggested that perhaps a Valium would help me sleep. I didn't take that too well because I feel that I have enough drugs in my system and deeply want to address my own fears and concerns by knowledge, confrontation, and good emotional management. He has been under a lot of stress and his natural reaction is to be less sensitive and more controlling out of pure frustration. He perceives that he knows what would be good for me in almost every situation and is upset when I don't go along with the program. It makes me feel pressure and even when I am following every suggestion, it is never quite enough to get the job done. So I ended up getting out my Walkman and listening to Crosby, Stills and Nash in the quiet of the night. I heard harmony and individual tracks I had never heard before even though I have listened to that tape no less than a thousand times. It was eerie. So I started to settle down a bit, on my own, without the damned Valium.

November 20th
I am finally out of bed at noon after a miserable night with a stomach virus.

Although I am irritated that I got it at all, I seem to be recovering faster than mere mortals who are not, after all, on chemotherapy white-blood-cell-killing treatment. I am going to do everything in my power to be well enough to take the hit of chemo #2 tomorrow.

Miraculously my hair held on for the company picnic. I think it was sheer willpower, as it was really trying to make a move. One of my golf buddies asked if I was ready to play golf. I said I didn't even know if I could swing the club. He went to his car and brought out his nine iron for me to see how it would feel. I agreed to try to play the following morning.

I stopped after nine holes but did pretty darned well considering that it was exactly six weeks and one day after the surgery on my chest. I wore a tennis hat pulled down over my head so I wouldn't have to deal with the hair problem. By this time, I couldn't even brush it or I wouldn't have any left. A gust of wind could actually blow it right off my head. So my hat was holding my hair on.

When I got home, I pulled the hat off and my hair was in it. I ran my hand across my head and more huge gobs came out. This was it. I stepped into my bathroom, seated myself on the floor in front of the toilet and proceeded to pull as much of it out by hand as I could. As I did so, pure hysterical emotion came pouring out and I just cried harder and harder, pulling and pulling, almost completely filling the toilet with my new wavy short hair.

Mark arrived and I closed the door before he got to me, refusing to come out, continuing to cry, feeling so ashamed. He stayed on the other side of the door patiently begging me to let him share. I just couldn't. I asked him to awaken Andrew and bring him to me. I thought he would find something to say to make it not so bad. He was just offbeat enough to find something cool in it.

He sat on the floor with me and let me cry on his broad, bare shoulder. He also had tears in his eyes but said that it would be okay. I said, "Look, all my hair is in the toilet. What am I going to do?" He replied "Get one of those wigs like the chick in Pulp Fiction!" Like, no big deal. An opportunity even. I was persuaded out of the bathroom and Mark took over. He set up the buzz razor that he used to cut the boys' hair. He buzzed all of the remaining clumps until I had no hair on my head at all. I was so traumatized that I was trembling and could not even find a way to lift my head to look in the mirror. Mark continually told me that it was beautiful, that I was beautiful, that he loved it and I would learn to also. Then he took my hand and placed it between his legs. He was excited.

Later that evening, Pete came home, being noisy and with something of an attitude. On a hunch, I dragged myself out of bed and joined him downstairs at a little after midnight where he was halfheartedly watching television. We sat and talked until 215 am, long overdue, shed some tears together and finally said some things that we had not been able to say since the whole thing started. He was sensitive and lovely and shared that just witnessing me and my attitude and the changes I had made, had allowed him to make similar changes in his own life, loosening up, taking a few more chances, being a little less tight with money, purchasing some items he was really enjoying. He even admitted t-p-ing a girlfriend's house that evening and having blown off a vocabulary test the week before. I told him that was fine but not to go overboard. He laughed. He seemed most concerned that we weren't telling him everything because he was totally counting on me to get well after the hospitalization and was just considering this current period "no big deal." Sort of like having the flu. I assured him it was a bigger deal than that but also assured him that I would get well and would not leave him. We were both smiling when we said good night and I slept great after that.

I am faring quite well with no hair actually. It is a very sensual experience in the shower and when a breeze comes over me. Life feels simple and focused in some ways, enormously complicated in others.

CHAPTER SIXTY-ONE

Even though my white cell count is still low, Dr. John says we will go ahead with the second chemo treatment and introduce a daily home injection of white cell stimulants for the next fourteen days. The cost of the round of shots is over a thousand dollars and I imagine the insurance company is starting to think of me as one of those cases that I know, as a business owner, make premiums skyrocket.

We are taught how to administer the shots in various places. Mark always lets me choose where I want it, depending on my mood. I alternate between my stomach and both thighs. He is very methodical and precise about it, inspiring confidence. During the fourteen days, my bones feel very busy. They buzz with activity and I see small white dots dancing about. Dr. John is amused by this, saying he has never heard of such "side effects," but admits that the purpose of the treatment is to kick-start production of cells in my bone marrow and that sounds suspiciously like what I am describing. The sensation doesn't scare me. It fills me with confidence that the treatment is working and I am delighted to know that my bones are becoming an ally in the fight against my disease. While I have always had a close connection to my physical self as a dancer, I have never experienced this level of awareness. It is thrilling.

The second chemo treatment is much more unpleasant and

difficult than the first. Still trying to avoid having a catheter surgically inserted, I get stuck every time and my veins are already beginning to break down. I am poked more than once this time and even when the needle finds the vein, it has to be manipulated inside the vein to make the connection. The anti-nausea drug makes me dizzy, and it is hard to believe it is working anyway considering the level of nausea I am experiencing. I remember early on thinking, *Well, how bad can nausea really be? I can handle that.* I now know that nausea can be extremely debilitating. In fact, chemo induced nausea should actually have a different name than the kind of nausea caused by the flu or a stomach ache or eating something that doesn't agree with you. They are not the same. Not even close.

Chemo enhances my ability to smell. I can walk in the front door and identify the strawberries sitting on the counter in the kitchen at the far end of the house. Sometimes I don't feel like eating at all, which makes me feel worse actually, so I am encouraged to eat pretty much anything that appeals to me on the theory that something in my stomach is better than nothing.

The drugs make my insides feel very claustrophobic. We take our little red convertible to Mayo for treatment because the fresh air on the ride home with the top down reduces the feeling of smothering inside.

CHAPTER SIXTY-TWO

It starts with a little plan I am brewing up to look for good fares to DC and hop a plane to treat myself to a visit. Underneath I am feeling lost at times, floating above and beyond those around me, wanting to be quiet and isolated. I feel I can do that with Michael without having to be alone and it is why I am drawn to the idea of visiting. It is his "knowing" everything about me and how I am thinking and feeling without words. I cling to that and wish it were more available to me. While the distance is difficult, it doesn't stop us from deepening our connection. In fact, it seems to enhance it, teaching us how to use our "other way" to communicate that does not require a fax, a phone, a computer, or a pen. He writes to me:

I cannot tell you enough how each moment of my life is spent with you. I carry you inside me and your breath travels alongside mine. It is you and your ability to embrace life and meaning that makes all this possible. It is something you have always had but has only recently been allowed to surface. Your sensitivity and understanding, the feelings you have inside, the care you feel for yourself and others, the natural way you have, all of these things are what make you the gift you are. You are unique and this quality seems to grow more so as we progress. You enhance my life and many others. I love you so much for it.

After I brew up that plan, I cook up another, far more legitimate, although cloaked in the guise of an excuse to get what I need. I want Michael to document what is happening to me. There is no one else I can possibly trust to photograph me in such a vulnerable state. It seems a necessary piece of my healing, a belief that maybe if we can make art of the whole thing, it won't be so scary. And if I don't survive, I will leave behind this haunting proof of who I was. It seems vitally important.

I present the idea to Mark one evening while we are out to dinner. He is supportive and even proud of me, acknowledging that it could be a bold, artistic statement. He actually expresses concern as to whether Michael can handle it emotionally, already knowing first hand how difficult it is to be the witness. I find it fascinating that he doesn't worry about my state of mind, thinking I am strong enough to endure such an experience. He gives his blessing. I buy a warm coat, gloves, and a hat to cover my bald head.

My friend Vicky finally finds the courage to walk away from the disastrous sexual relationship with her priest and move to North Carolina. She tells me of an intuitive memory about a doctor who wrote a book about cancer and feels I must have it. The doctor is Bernie Siegel and the book, Love, Medicine and Miracles. I am convinced in the scheme of the universe that he wrote it just for me and once I read it, I carry it around for two weeks, never letting it out of my sight. He believes in a community of what he calls "exceptional cancer patients" and I know I am one of those. The book is filled with stories of the deep symbolism of cancer. Once that symbolism is discovered and embraced, miraculous healing can occur, far beyond the obvious. Other than my immediate family, he is the first person to validate that sexual abuse is my cancer and by destroying it, the effects of the abuse will be destroyed as well. I believe it completely and contact Dr. Siegel to let him know how right he is. He calls me back and we begin a wonderful correspondence. His message is always the same. Find a creative outlet for what you are going through. Keep a journal, write poetry, paint, or dance. I already know he is right. I am so grateful to my friend for knowing I need Bernie. She sends me a prayer:

> *Be at peace. Do not look forward in fear to the changes of life. Rather look to them with full hope as they arise. God, whose very own you are, will deliver you from out of them. He has kept you hitherto and will lead you safely through all things; and when you cannot stand it, God will bury you in his arms. Do not fear what may happen tomorrow. The same everlasting Father who cares for you today will take care of you then and every day. He will either shield you from suffering or will give you unfailing strength to bear it. Be at peace and put aside all anxious thoughts and imaginations.*

I invite her to meet Michael and me at a museum in Virginia, about halfway between where she lives and where we will be in DC, while I am visiting. She agrees. It will be great to see her.

CHAPTER SIXTY-THREE

I fly off to DC to have my picture made. Michael has recommended a wonderful old hotel in the District where I have a suite. Once an apartment building, my room has a kitchen, a big living room, a bedroom and an old fashioned bathroom with an intricately patterned black and white tile floor. There is a fold-out couch in the front room where Michael sleeps. He can't bring himself to go home each night and leave me alone.

I have gone over and over in my mind what it will be like for him to see me with no hair. I am sure his only concern is taking care of me and taking the photographs I have requested but I worry just the same. I feel so exposed and raw going to him that only the extraordinary degree of trust that exists between us can protect me from being destroyed by simply being looked at. Looked through, because I feel transparent, like all my organs and cells and feelings and weaknesses and fears are on display. Actually, to Michael, they are.

We sit on the couch and I won't take off my scarf in front of him. He doesn't push me but reaches over gently to slide off the bandana slowly and with great care. His hands rub and caress my bald head while I close my eyes, tears escaping down my cheeks. He tells me repeatedly that my head is beautiful and I am beautiful. I feel okay after that, able to be completely open with myself in his presence.

He shoots pictures constantly. Mostly black and white. When I sit in the big chair in the living room after coming back from dinner, he shoots me in my short skirt, black turtleneck and heels after I have just pulled the pretty silk scarf off my head and it is draped over my lap. He shoots me in the morning before I can find the energy to get up out of bed, head still on the pillow, feeling so poorly. He shoots me as I prepare the syringe for the shots that he gives me even though he is terrified of needles. He shoots me from overhead while I am taking a bath and also while my chin is resting on the edge of the tub, beads of moisture all over my face. He is so quiet and subtle with his task that I feel completely comfortable allowing whatever my feelings are to surface, not worrying in the least about the camera, which may as well be invisible. I am relieved to send my intense feelings somewhere else, especially to a place where they can be examined later. How very much I believe I can learn from that.

One day we go to his art studio. I put on my jeans, bandana and dangly earrings, and we walk over from the hotel. Dance bag over my shoulder, "costumes" in the bag, it feels like I am going to a performance, a sensation that reminds me of confident and beloved times in my past. It is cold when we arrive. I put on dance clothes and begin to feel traumatized at the prospect of what we are about to do. Not because I am shy about being photographed or reluctant to go through with it but because I know that I am going to meet my disease face to face in this process, actually see it for the first time. While Michael sets up, I sit quietly on the floor in front of the plain grey backdrop. I bury my head in my arms, contemplating what it will be like to go this far into myself and wondering what I will find there. He captures that image, unbeknownst to me. He shoots a set of black and white Polaroids to test the light and keeps pulling them off the camera. Finally he asks if I want to see them and lays them out in a circle on the floor around me. I am stunned by what I see in my own face, things that are not visible in the mirror. Every emotion I am feeling or have felt since I made my tumor is right there in each photograph. I am shocked but somehow relieved and commit fully to the process at hand, unable to hide my intense emotion even if I wanted to. I take most of my clothes off for some shots, all of them for others, forcing myself to confront my battered body for the lens, coming to terms with it. I am cold and in between set-ups he puts his long wool coat over my shoulders. He shoots me in nothing but the coat with bare feet. The images that come out of the professional box camera are mostly the ones that later will be exhibited, but I still love the Polaroids. They are the most intimate, the most personal, the most raw, the most honest.

Before I leave, we drive to Richmond to meet Vicky, as planned. She seems disturbed that I am so completely involved with Michael and that he is so protective of me in every way. She finds it inappropriate and mentions it directly to both of us in the context of Mark and what she perceives we are really up to. It leaves me feeling unsettled and off balance.

Later she calls Mark and voices her observations and concerns. They speak on the phone for well over an hour. I know this only when I see the charge on our phone bill later. But it explains why, while I am gone, he breaks a double lock on my desk drawer at the office and takes my journal and letters and faxes. This includes everything I have written about my behavior with James, the unabridged version, as well as everything that has passed between me and Michael in the past year. When he picks me up at the airport, he will have read it all. No more secrets.

The morning that Michael has to say goodbye and leave me in my room, I panic. I don't want him to go and can't bear the thought of it. He comforts me as I cry hysterically and beg him to stay but we both know he has to go. When he walks out of the room, the cleaning lady, who has obviously heard my cries, gives him a very disapproving look which is devastating to him. The staff has adopted me during my short stay. They don't ask me about what I am going through, just take good care of me, anticipating my every need and treating me with such kindness. They make me promise to make the Hotel Lombardy my permanent home in Washington DC and to this day, it is.

My friend, Frankie, whose family was stationed with us in Holland and is my oldest friend, arrives to save the day a few hours later, unaware of my emotional state. He comes up to my room and hugs me so hard I can't breathe and I think he may never let go. We have breakfast downstairs and head to Annapolis for the day. The drive is beautiful. It is cold and crisp and gorgeous on the water and I am bundled up with a beautiful, soft, warm scarf around my neck that Michael gave me. We stroll through the quaint village and I buy a homemade Christmas ornament, a lighthouse. We have a wonderful lunch at an Italian place with a big fire burning. I share a select group of the Polaroids with him. He is totally blown away and at one point, excuses himself to go to the bathroom. I follow to the ladies' room and I can hear him blowing his nose. I am sure he is crying and doesn't want me to see.

On the way to the airport, he takes my hand and holds it all the way there. When he drops me and my bags at the curb, he hugs me and kisses me three times and cries real tears. He is so emotional, thanks me again for sharing the photographs, saying he will remember me. I know he regrets that comment under the circumstances but I know what he really means.

And so I board the plane to go home. I write to Michael:

You were so sensitive and supportive and loving to me, it broke my heart. What an incredible feeling to trust so much. I don't know how to express my feelings about these past few days but I take heart in knowing you that already know everything. It is sad to part and is, for a brief time, totally unbearable. But we take so many wonderful things away with us that will enrich our lives. And my heart is full of love and joy and peace. And with that comes healing. You have been a brilliant guide along the way as you have an incredible capacity to give love unconditionally. In my life, I never expected to experience such an amazing gift and I feel blessed.

Mark is waiting for me at the gate.

CHAPTER SIXTY-FOUR

Mark waits until I am settled from the trip, comes into my office, closes the door behind him, and confronts me with the evidence he has collected while I was gone. At the same time, Michael is receiving a fax from Mark at his office. He plans it so that both Michael and I will be surprised at virtually the exact same moment and cannot confer with each other in advance.

Dear Michael,

Thank you for your kind support of Trish during these difficult times.

The evolution of relationships can be an interesting process. Seldom is it unfettered by constraints and circumstances which impinge on the free flow of that process—although we try sometimes to ignore them. Indeed, the most efficacious and sophisticated method of ignoring impediments to a relationship developing in a desired fashion is to first acknowledge them, and then reject them by means of rationalization, justification, and minimization. The door opens to indulgence in the cherished and sought after feelings, emotions, and behaviors. Half admit. Be half honest. Trish has become expert in this regard. A little truth can obscure a lot of truth. I am not in a position to fully measure your adroitness regarding this technique, but I suspect it is at least adequate.

The point being, the relationship between you and Trish has escalated over the past couple years to a plateau which is, with my concept of marriage—my marriage, certainly—incompatible.

For what it's worth — as blame becomes an irrelevant concept — I attach very little of it to you, less and less to Trish, and more to myself for not recognizing this pattern of hers as an addiction and dealing with it accordingly.

As you probably know — at least as much as she wanted you to know — Trish was ending what can only be described as — because of, at the very least, the intense emotional intimacy involved — an affair with a man she was infatuated with initially some twenty-odd years ago. Simultaneously with that end, it appears that your rekindled relationship and connections intensified, also achieving some months prior to this writing and continuing to this day, an extraordinarily high degree of intimacy. Again, whether you or Trish choose to acknowledge it as such, the two of you are conducting — in some ways different than the preceding one, but in all essential ways the same — an affair.

You give to Trish prodigious amounts of what she says she wants and needs. Glibness is not intended when I ask you, If a junkie asked you for twenty bucks to get a fix, would you give it to him? Yes, and it hurts me to reduce it to this but I seriously have come to believe — and I have been dealing with this for years and years, Michael — that it is addiction with which we are dealing. She is addicted not just to the feelings and passions and emotions but also to the secrecy; the clandestine letters, faxes, conversations, voice mail messages, trips. ..all of it. And it is no less powerful than alcohol, cocaine, heroin, sex, power, or any other addiction.

I wallowed through the previous "affair", not understanding until recently the degree and intensity of it. Had I understood then, I would not have tolerated it; nor do I intend to tolerate this one, understanding what I do now. Trish's probable representation to you that I was fine with and supported her throughout the James debacle was only partially true, premised on a very distorted reality provided to me by her; and fostered by a misunderstanding, I now believe, of the underlying dynamics. And quite frankly, she is repeating the distortion of having also misrepresented your relationship—thereby allowing me to support it as well. Bits and pieces of the truth to cover the lie.

I suppose if I were allowed to have my cake and eat it too, it would be difficult not to indulge. Trish has effectively challenged that well-tested axiom with, I'm afraid, some complicity on my part and considerable success on hers—but only if success is measured on a very superficial plane and without balancing it against its considerable cost to others and to herself. She believes that she can obtain certain things only by operating outside the boundaries of her marriage. That is simply the fallacy which shelters the addiction. And ultimately the deception, the secrets, the duplicity; along with the drug of intimacy with men, men other than her husband—and you are not singular in that regard—are the poisons eating away at her very self. There exists no balance, delicate or otherwise.

Perhaps in this instance as regards most old saws, there resides some fundamental truth. Perhaps it would be better to choose rather than challenge the conventional wisdom; better to have one or to do the other; better to meet head-on the true challenge which is neither sexual abuse nor cancer. It is not about her "rights" or what she "deserves" or what she was "denied" or "lost". It is about her marriage, and the importance it has in her life.

Perhaps I will stage a one-man "intervention" as is done with addicts of all kinds at which she will surely argue that she needs these things; among them your "love" and affections, your sensitivities and sensibilities and attentions, the kindness and understanding (all those things for which some reason still beyond my grasp I am held to be inadequate) only you (or some other man besides me) can provide, and that she needs them desperately to be healed; and I will argue my proposition that those are exactly the things from which she needs to free herself to heal. And then I suppose all sorts of choices will present themselves—to both of us.

And choices are hard. I know. I'm making my own. I'm trying to find a place in this that is right for me, you see. So far in these matters I have not really had "my place" but rather the place Trish has assigned to me, and I am not comfortable with that, and I choose not to accept it any longer. I am quite tired of her conducting her affairs—which in essence have a very "fantastic," fantasy-like, unreal, image-on-the-screen-like quality—and then returning to our very real life and relationship and asking me to measure up to the standards and behaviors and attentions—derived from that "unreal" context—of other men.

I suggest you and Trish get together and decide exactly how you intend to resolve this. I am not opposed to honest, sincere, friendship and affection, if that can be accomplished (although I do suspect it's hard to make an advancing glacier recede). And, of course, in the beginning, that's what it "appeared" to be and at a conscious level probably was; and she told me about it, and of course, I had no objection at all. But she never reveals the changes, the escalations, the complications, the ultimate intimacy, grotesquely applying my original compliance to everything that follows.

And I know you are an honorable and sincere man possessing no conscious intention to do harm to anyone. But is it possible your own needs and desires have overwhelmed clarity? And Trish has provided you a "version" of her life—a very careful construct of her life and our relationship—designed specifically to allow you (and her) to justify your relationship as being all right, permissible, appropriate. (I think she did that with James, too, although it was more for herself than for him. I don't think he cared. I believe you do. This time the facade is for both of you.) Has not your better judgment suffered?

But fair warning. I have no doubt that what you give to her is something she wants (must have?) very much. And if you and she are convinced that it is a genuine quality, an essential part of a "healthy Trish" and not an addiction, and does not and should not be tempered or "treated"--and you're all she has--what you have to give will very soon not be nearly enough.

I am overcome by a multitude of emotions, forced to deal with the consequences of what got me into this mess in the first place. Mark is angry and hurt. He has completely exposed my inner life. The secret place where I live with James, Michael, and the residue of sexual abuse. I resent the intrusion into my privacy, and particularly detest the cold, logical tone of his letter that I feel should be a more emotional statement. This just underscores my belief that he can never understand the passion of James or the artistic tenderness of Michael. But I somehow trust his instinct to confront, even at such a difficult time in the middle of my treatment. He sits in the bathroom with me as I am bathing, demanding to know exactly what happened on my trip, how far it has gone with Michael. I won't discuss such details, needing to keep them private, and he retreats. Of course, my pre-cancer journal has delivered every sexual detail about James and I am only beginning to process the impact of that knowledge. Gradually I begin to feel the incredible relief of what my husband has done, what I would never have been able to do for myself.

CHAPTER SIXTY-FIVE

It is the Christmas season and oddly, it is the most stress-free holiday I have ever experienced. Cancer creates a perfect bubble in which to exist filled with many special privileges and advantages. No one expects me to go out and do my usual shopping. So I give each of the boys the same amount of money, tell them to buy exactly what they most want, wrap everything in pretty paper, and place it all under the tree so I can have the pleasure of watching them open their gifts on Christmas morning. I am treated with great care at home, at the office, and wherever I go since it is quite obvious that I am a cancer patient. People speak to me in public and share their stories. It is not always easy to hear about their loved ones who didn't make it, but I try to be kind and responsive. I am offended by those who complain about having a bad hair day or not wishing to celebrate yet another birthday because they are getting too old. I tell my employees who smoke in our office courtyard that if they could just experience one round of chemotherapy, they would never smoke again.

Christmas means a week off from the chemo cycle to collect my stem cells and put them in the freezer until they are needed for the transplant. I will require a surgically placed catheter under my collarbone, a stiff one to accommodate a free flow of blood in and out of the machine that will extract my stem cells.

I go into pre-op not really understanding what is involved. It is described as relatively minor, in and out kind of thing, especially for a thin person like me because the great vein is easier to find in this blind procedure. An x-ray machine is used to help the surgeon place the wire and then the catheter over it. A very clumsy resident, an assistant to the surgeon, comes over to disclose the risks and secure my consent. First he says that they could slip and collapse a lung and other terrifying possibilities at which point he says that saying these things to patients only "scares them to death" but he is required to do so. Then he asks me if "they" have told me where they want this catheter, which does not fill me with confidence. (Funny, I am thinking he should know.) I tell him "they" pointed to the collarbone area but I assume it is up to the surgeon to know these things. Then a wonderful anesthesia nurse named Faith comes to me with a giant hypodermic needle filled with my "tonic." I ask what it is and she says something like Valium and there will be more of that and a narcotic in the operating room later. I ask if it is optional and she says yes so I refuse it, stating that I think the local anesthesia will be fine. She says that if I change my mind at any time I can let her know and she will open the IV. Someone probably should have mentioned that it is not just an anxiety sedative but instead numbs the intense pain of a sharp, stiff, fat object being forced into your great vein. (Like being harpooned, the nurse says later.)

I get wheeled into an operating room and still have not seen the real surgeon when I am draped over my face. I explain that I would like to see him in person before the procedure begins. He appears and is very nice and talks to me but then allows the clumsy resident to actually perform the procedure. (*Hey, buddy. This isn't an episode of ER. This is real life. My life,* I want to say. *Do the damned procedure yourself. Let him practice on someone else. I've got a transformation to get to.*) When he begins to push clumsily into that vein, intense pain shoots up my neck and all the way down my arm. I practically jump off the table and tell them as calmly as I can that I am definitely experiencing the radiating pain up into my neck they said I should immediately tell them about if it occurs. Very agitated now, I am losing control of the situation. The pain is so searing that passing out cold is the only way I can imagine that it can be tolerated. I try levitating, which I am certain I must actually be doing. They decide it is too late to stop to adjust pain medication now that they are "in" and because I am so verbal now, I'm guessing they think they better keep hearing from me to monitor my considerable distress rather than knock me out, while I am thinking that is such a merciful idea. Under great duress, the young surgeon finally gets the large, stiff catheter into place and the nurse assures me that it is pretty much over. She looks like she has just seen a ghost.

Later I discover that the nurses were practically in tears witnessing my overwhelming pain and one was ready with more anesthetic in her hand repeatedly urging the resident to use it although he never gave the order. The nurses stay with me in recovery and are concerned. I am learning that it's what nurses do sometimes. Clean up the mess.

Even though it is tough going cold turkey like that on the procedure, I think it is a real benefit for the next day during the stem cell collection as I will not have to deal with the extended effects of the narcotics in my system to which I am very sensitive. I can't bear the idea of collecting my stem cells while under the influence of some drug. I have considerable discomfort throughout the night, able only to lie flat on my back because the catheter is several inches long and cannot be crunched. Instead my shoulder has to remain flat and stable. It is so close to my lung that anything more than a small breath causes discomfort.

CHAPTER SIXTY-SIX

Exactly one week before Christmas Eve, I am scheduled to spend a minimum of four mornings in a row at the Blood Bank for pheresis, the technical name for collection of stem cells. I am feeling very debilitated when I arrive, shaky and worn out from the difficult experience of having my catheter installed the day before. A nice fellow named Kyle starts by taking my blood pressure and telling me not to worry. The procedure, says Kyle, is "boring and benign." I tease him mercilessly about his choice of the benign word. My pressure is so low, he can't even get a reading. Not a good sign. Kyle looks a little concerned, through a warm smile.

The idea is to send all the blood in and out of my body through the machine three times, extracting the stem cells as we go. There are needles in both arms making me a perfect circle of movement. During the four hours plus procedure, I turn beautiful shades of yellow and green, throw up, get very dizzy, nauseous, and shake like a leaf. I am covered by several blankets and a heating pad and attended to by some of the most wonderful, kindest people I have ever encountered. The third hour is particularly tough when I seem to just run out of steam. But the collection is excellent quality. I can see that for myself as I look at the lovely, vibrant small bag of stem cells we have accumulated. My caretakers are very pleased, amazed even. It is exhausting but judging from their response, it seems I am overachieving.

When the work is done, I am desperately hungry. There is an urgency to it that cannot be described, like everything I used to have inside me is now in the bag on its way to the freezer. Mark rushes me to the nearest Mexican restaurant where I inhale the biggest, most filling meal I can possibly eat.

And then we go back and do it again the next day. And the next. They almost cancel the fourth day, saying they actually have enough from the first two collections to use for the transplant, which is very unusual. But we go ahead anyway, just to make sure. I guess when you are about to destroy your immune system, you can never have enough stem cells in the freezer. Just in case.

I write a letter to the doctor in charge of the Blood Bank:

The blessings associated with my cancer experience have been many and strangely, I wouldn't change places at this moment with my old "healthy" self, even knowing what I still have to face. How odd that cancer will save my life.

Among the many blessings that have presented themselves to me is the realization that the world is full of wonderful, dedicated, caring people such as those that work at United Blood Services. In my old life, it did not seem necessary to depend on anyone. But now, depending on those who provide my medical care is a necessity, one to which I have had to adjust. That trust is not given easily and your staff certainly gained it the old-fashioned way. They earned it.

Admittedly, I was a bit traumatized by facing this procedure partly because it seemed to be the first actual step toward the stem cell rescue, making it finally seem real. That meant facing a lot of fear about the future.

Kyle put me immediately at ease and committed himself fully to not only the success of the procedure but my continuing comfort. It did not take me long to feel confident in that relationship allowing me to give more and more of myself along the way. And then I had the pleasure of getting to know the rest of the staff. The grinding energy of Pete, who never seems to lose sight of what he is there for. The quiet knowledge and concern of Anita who always seemed to be there when I needed a reassuring look. And, of course, the running monologue pouring out of Sam while she is providing extremely competent, confidence-inspiring care. And your personal attention on a daily basis was deeply appreciated. I enjoyed our chats very much.

I find that I cannot resist relating a few moments that fondly stand out in my mind. The sheer panic on Kyle's very available face when I announced that I was going to throw "up" and, unable to immediately find something in which for me to do it, he picked up the large, half-full trash can and placed it in the air over my face. Despite my concern about attempting to throw up leaning back in the chair with a trash can upside down over my face, I was able to lean forward and he was able to locate a clean trash bag for the episode. We all laughed about it after. My unfortunate announcement that I had to get unhooked yet one more time to go to the bathroom much to the dismay of my family members and others, looking beyond all their faces and seeing Anita mouthing the words "It's okay" to me. Watching Ruth work like a busy bee at her little desk the whole time but on one occasion coming to me concerned about whether my hands were cold. She put together two hot water bottles and brought them to me which helped tremendously. (I doubt that particular behavior is in her job description.) The West side "floater," Virginia, making a point of introducing herself to me and checking in each day to see how I was doing, sometimes taking a few moments to share Mom stories. A big hug from Marilyn upon my departure on Wednesday. A somber and sincere message from Pete as he stopped by my chair between visits to the field telling me how much they would be praying for me as I faced the next part of the procedure, hoping it would go as well as this one had.

Please share this letter with your staff and accept my best wishes for a wonderful Christmas and a joyous and happy New Year. I myself am planning many more, in part thanks to you.

CHAPTER SIXTY-SEVEN

All energy is now pointed towards the February transplant, stem cell rescue, spiritual rebirth. I relish the rescue/rebirth part, not the procedure part. By then, I will be ready. I have put on weight since the stem cell collection took so much out of me, literally. I am back in the gym. Training.

Vicky terminates our relationship by letter, stating it has become toxic to her. I am devastated. Mark, in his constant state of grace, patiently helps me understand that the letter is about Vicky, not me. I know it is about sexual abuse and its collateral damage. We throw it away and move on. He says I don't need her or anyone to get well. He's right. I'm okay.

Submitting to chemo #3 is easier, partly due to experience and attitude and partly due to the two-week out of cycle break during stem cell collection allowing me more recovery time. I can't believe this is happening. I learn to take it one day at a time. I sleep better, deeper, later. I feel enormous peace and joy and that is a brilliant surprise at a time like this.

January 9th
I felt blue this morning, edgy and emotional. Day 14 of chemo, everything bottoming out. Last shot burned and hurt like crazy. I was hard on Mark for no reason. He felt bad.

We tour the transplant unit. Our guide, the manager, is very impressive. The nurses seem wonderful, and the rooms are sunny with treadmills and stationary bikes, clean filtered air and VCR's. I admit to being scared but she says I can influence my own progress with determination and attitude.

My white cells are stellar. The shots are working. I am still seeing stars and my bones are buzzing.

I talk to Michael on the phone. There is a big blizzard in Washington DC that has shut down the entire area. He walks three miles to the Metro station to get into the city to work. He's been shoveling for days, assisting neighbors. I love his comment that while walking three miles in the freezing cold, he knows he should feel cranky but just can't because it is so breathtakingly beautiful. I would give anything for a major weather change. A storm. Besides the one going on inside of me.

January 10th
I am afraid I am losing my eyebrows and lashes. A few seem to be letting loose. I hope not. I am being very careful with them. If I can just hang on until the hospital, then everything will start to grow again. I hope, I hope.

January 23rd
Stomach is screaming. Body is shaking.

February 1st
I felt real good when I got home last night, very relieved, happy and peaceful but with the same sadness that is always there, still there. Pete came down later in the evening and threw his head on my lap and lamented that a nasty teacher of his had stuck them with learning all the Latin American countries on the map as well as all the capitals plus 25 vocabulary words for a quiz the following day. He

was overwhelmed. So he came up to my room where we snuck a look at Seinfeld while attempting to figure out creative ways to remember those capitals. Instead of succeeding, we just made silly jokes and laughed until we were crazy. Then we collapsed into giving turns, four minutes each, two-minute back scratch and two minute back of the legs. That felt so good we had to repeat the turns, only this time I got a special head rub, and those capitals just kept fading away from our memories. We considered, of course, staying under the covers all day and just playing hooky from quizzes and work but Mark discouraged that. Cooler heads prevailed. Peter is so big now with such long arms and legs that he hardly fits on the bed along with Jill, the coyote dog. I love the crowded feeling of having them both with me. Mark is annoyed by it, doesn't really participate, and wants it all to be over so he can go to sleep. So we just ignore him. We finally gave it up and went to bed. I had a nice sleep until 430 am. Then it got very crowded inside of me.

I make the mistake of failing to prepare properly for my fourth and final outpatient chemo treatment. Thinking I am an old pro by now, I sail into it without the mental and emotional work necessary to stay one step ahead of how terrible it is. So it has its way with me and I am sick as a dog until I bottom out two weeks later. Two miserable weeks.

Finally things begin to move in the opposite direction. My face is brightening up. I have come to love the feeling of enduring the wrath of a chemo treatment, riding it down to the darkest point, and then feeling the good cells begin to take over, regenerate, and slowly bring me back to life. It fills me with hope that in a bigger sense, I can accomplish the same thing. Ride my disease to the darkest places inside of me and slowly bring myself back to life, whole and clean. That is the work that lies ahead of me now.

Mark and I, still licking our respective wounds, continue to work things out. This morning he heats lotion in the heating pad and instructs me to take a long, hot shower. He does, too. He gives me a long, full body lotion rub and much, much more. He is sweet and loving with no anger or attitude. It is so wonderful, peaceful and healing. I cry.

He orders the Spice channel for us later. It is hilariously rank. But fun.

I spend time with Andrew and Peter, telling them not to consider frequent hospital visits an obligation. We watch a funny animated TV show called Dr. Katz and I laugh. Andrew says he hasn't heard me laugh in a while.

I enjoy a wonderful lunch with Peter. He says he will hide me out if I change my mind about the transplant or we can just keep going and drive straight to Coronado Island instead. Whatever I want. I laugh until I am silly. Great medicine, great joy.

I tell Michael that if he comes to get me soon, I can skip the transplant. He says that other than my own family, no one will ever love me more than he does.

Mark and I treat ourselves to dinner at our favorite expensive restaurant. The food is remarkable. Lobster ravioli, grilled Maine lobster with lemon dill pasta, raspberry tart with hot tea.

Pete goes with me to pick out a CD Walkman and some new music for the hospital. Then we have fries. This time next week I will be half way through high dose chemo.

I feel so much love. People send cards and hug me and wish me well. I know that is because there is grave concern that I won't even survive the transplant. But I feel their prayers and well wishes and it means a lot. I feel cherished.

I take care of last minute office details in preparation for my long absence from work. I get another lotion rub and head straight to the airport. Mark and I have determined it would be good for me to spend one night at the shore to get ready for what is ahead. I board a not crowded plane to San Diego, my beloved Coronado. Mark encourages me to upgrade my room when I get there to full ocean view at the Hotel del Coronado. Maybe I will.

CHAPTER SIXTY-EIGHT

My beautiful sixth floor room in the Ocean Tower has a big, soft bed with huge throw pillows, a striped couch and a pretty armchair. The oceanfront side is ceiling to floor glass and I keep the curtains and door open at all times. While waiting to get into my room, I have my traditional roast beef on French roll, Pepsi and chips on the Ocean Terrace. It is a brilliant, sunny day and the sky is deep blue. I take a long walk to my usual spot on the sand hill by our summer condo next door to the hotel, rubbing blisters on my feet. I take off my scarf and feel the ocean breeze on my skull. Back at the hotel, a charming sparrow actually flies into my room.

I have a vision, a waking dream. It is incredible, unforgettable. My go-ahead sign. A globe floating in space. A large, white hand appears from the left, holding a turtle. It looks like the hand of God, powerful, strong and loving. The turtle is active, curious, happy, with arms and legs swimming and head fully extended. The hand is placing the turtle on the world. It's God giving me back to the earth, fully out of my shell.

Then on to Prima Vera for dinner at the bar, my favorite place to hang out when I am alone at the shore, where I consider the staff to be friends. I am eating a brilliant plate of food, nervous about where Michael's sister, Judy and her husband Lex will position themselves and why they are so insistent on coming so far to see me and why I am taking my precious private time to talk kids and suburbs. Four terrific hours later, I know exactly why. Judy is so like Michael, looks exactly like him, talks like him, cares like him. I feel his presence there with us. Lex is talkative and very interested in things. When I ask him, as a PhD cancer research scientist, what he knows about stem cell rescues, he says it will tax me mentally and physically, will be very tough. I panic and spend the next two hours talking to him about my perspective, experience, the Mayo Clinic, my ability to endure and most of all, my belief that it is my fate. At the end of the evening, after I show him Michael's photographs of me, he takes it back. I will do fine, he says, and the photos should become a book that belongs on the table of every waiting room of every breast clinic in the country. They later tell Michael they could have stayed all night talking, hating to leave.

The next morning, I have a wonderful talk with Judy on the phone sitting on my big bed overlooking the ocean. She tells me that, in Michael, I have been given an amazing gift. Accept it. It's unconditional. No need to take any baggage into my transplant. Just accept. Tearfully, I decide to take her advice. The ocean breeze finds me all the way into the shower. I have a wonderful breakfast on the balcony filled with the hypnotic power of the sea, and hope.

I take one last walk before I go. Standing on my favorite spot facing the ocean, where I have spent some of the happiest times of my life, I have a talk with God whose presence seems to fill the sky. I acknowledge the instant faith that appeared to me on the operating table during my biopsy, still growing and burning strong inside of me. I admit to being afraid but resolute in my unyielding desire to be well. I understand perfectly the opportunity I have been given for profound healing. I ask for the strength and grace to endure the physical challenge ahead. I promise that when my work is complete, I will take up the work for which I am being saved, whatever it is. God's investment in me will pay off. I promise.

It is Valentine's Day. I fly back after twenty-eight glorious hours at the shore. I'm ready.

CHAPTER SIXTY-NINE

Mark, Andrew, and Peter believe, individually and collectively, that I have gotten sick to get well and that no harm will come to me. (I guess that depends on your definition of harm but what they mean is they are sure that neither my disease, nor this procedure, will kill me.) Their strong certainty on the matter is a lifeline to which I cling, all the while constantly looking for some intuitive sign that it is really just a strategy that allows them the luxury of denial and they aren't really that certain at all. But no such sign appears. I come to believe that they truly believe what they say. There is a calmness, a power to their belief and gradually I choose to accept it as truth.

I must be very careful as to what influences to introduce into my sterile room. Dr. John has made it clear that I can only have one bone marrow transplant so whatever I am hoping to accomplish in my room, metaphysical or otherwise, must be done this time around. With Bernie Siegel as my mentor, I accept that what I am really doing is burning out the dark influences that were placed on me in my young life with high dose chemo and making a clean, new life for myself. This ultimately leads me to know for sure that my parents must not be allowed in my room during the procedure. So I ask Mark to accompany me to their home to break the news to them. I am extremely nervous, knowing how badly they will take it. I hold onto Mark's hand throughout and he helps me explain

Cancer again proves to be a protective blessing for me as they know they must be careful with their response considering I have cancer and am about to undergo a bone marrow transplant. So they don't argue too much. But it is obvious that they do not buy the theory of my disease, do not agree with my position, and immediately try to figure out how they are going to explain to everyone else in their lives why they are not by my bedside wearing masks and gowns. It makes keeping the family secret more difficult. They also figure out rather quickly that they do not have a say in the matter and I am determined. It feels like the first time I actually exercise the power my disease has afforded me.

The night before I enter the hospital, we go out to dinner as a family. We choose a nice restaurant and make a special occasion out of it. We agree that by the end of the evening, we will conduct a vote, a show of hands, as to whether I will actually report to the transplant the next day. In advance, it is determined that if any one of us does not vote in the positive, I will not have the procedure. I take it very seriously, pretending that the outcome is uncertain, that each vote including mine is still undecided, believing it is possible that I will cancel the whole thing. I cannot bear the thought that if something goes wrong, a motherless child will be left wondering why his voice wasn't heard. I want everyone completely invested. I want everyone to have a say. But it is clear that the other three, the Dutch boys, already know how they will vote and aren't giving it another thought. They're just enjoying the dinner. I am annoyed by this, thinking they are being somewhat cavalier about what I am about to endure. I practically have to remind them at the end of the dinner that we are there for the vote. It is unanimous. We're going for rebirth. How can they be so sure?

When everyone is asleep, except me, I slip out of bed and down the stairs, hoping it is not the last night I will ever spend in my home. I feel a burning need to review my life, not because I am afraid to die, but because it seems that my "rescue" will bring to a close the life I have lived so far. Maybe it is a need to honor that life, acknowledge it, and collect the memories so I may hold them close before I let them go. Let it all go in my sterile room.

I head to the University to visit the "Oasis," the first place I ever lived on my own and where I met Mark. It looks exactly the same. Close by is Gammage Auditorium which first lured me to Arizona State with its stunning architecture, where I stood in the sprinklers on that hot summer day twenty-five years ago, and where I had the great pleasure of performing many times. I look across the street to James' office where I held my life together by a thread. I can also see Lyric Opera Theatre, known as the Birthday Cake for its unusual round design, where I had my first professional choreography job and enjoyed performing in more than a dozen shows including the first one Mark attended. And I drive to the old Lyceum, the tiny theatre where I auditioned to get into the theatre degree program, and played Catherine in Henry V, entirely in French. I sit on the curb in front of my first dance studio with the beautiful big windows and the spring wood floor, only a short distance from our first townhouse where we lived when we married and when Andrew was born. Seeing our first real house just down the street makes me recall how thrilled we were with this beautiful, brand new two-story, complete with swimming pool in the back yard where Andrew learned to swim and pick up keys from the bottom of the pool when he could barely walk. Peter was conceived in this house and I used to walk him to the park by the lake under the moon late at night while he was still in my belly. All of these images help me remember who I am, especially the strong, healthy parts of me, the parts I want to take with me and integrate into the new.

Into this night I wander
It's morning that I dread
Another day of knowing of
The path I fear to tread
Oh into the sea of waking dreams
I follow without pride
Nothing stands between us here
And I won't be denied
—Sarah McLachlan

Sarah's words on the car stereo say what I already feel. Her images of dreading the morning, following without pride into the sea of waking dreams and refusing to be denied give me the luxury of not having to expend the energy to conceive of them myself. For that I am very grateful, just riding on the words safely, almost effortlessly. In some ways, it seems impossible that I find myself in this situation. In others, it seems like I have been waiting for it for such a long while. The impact of this little trip through my life is sobering, but it helps me put everything to rest and prepare for tomorrow. I return home and slip back into bed beside my husband and fall asleep.

CHAPTER SEVENTY

Friday morning is emotional for my employees as they bid me goodbye and wish me luck on my bone marrow transplant. I am feeling emotional, too, but not scared. Can't for the life of me figure out why not.

I go to Mayo around noon to have a pick line inserted into my left arm. It is a sterile procedure performed by a chemo nurse but they let Mark stay while wearing a mask. He may as well get used to it as he will spend a good part of the next month or so behind a mask in my sterile room. Nurse Judy is very serious and unbelievably competent but I make her laugh. She places a large needle in my vein with a long, soft catheter attached which has a guide wire in it so it can be pushed all the way up my vein towards my heart.

Later an x-ray confirms that it has landed in the right place and missed my jugular vein. That's good news! It takes a big dressing and is a bit bloody. Not too painful but already starting to feel sore.

Then on to outpatient surgery for placement of the Hickman catheter, which will provide two ports for chemo, medicine, drawing of blood etc., so I will no longer have to endure the needle stick each time. I luck out and get the gum-chewing, pearl-wearing, "junior high" surgeon, new to the staff, who looks to be not a day over sixteen. She is very smart and straightforward, concerned about my prior experience of severe pain during the first catheter placement when I opted for skipping the hard drugs. I figured it doesn't matter as much this time as many more drugs are to follow anyway. So what the hell?

She turns me over to dear Pauline, the Irish anesthetist nurse. We talk about my fear of being drugged and knocked out. So she keeps me awake until the hurt part and then nods me very gently off to sleep. I feel like she is holding me in her arms. When I awake, there is dear, sweet Pauline smiling at me with her kind Irish eyes and speaking to me in her beautiful brogue saying that it is over and all is well. (She goes on my angel list.) When I see Mark in recovery I cry a bit. He is overwhelmed now and prefers to concentrate on duties rather than emotion. I hope we can work on that during this time.

Upon arriving at the hospital, I am wheeled up to the Virginia Piper Bone Marrow Transplant Unit (like I can't walk) and introduced to my new home for the next few weeks. My cocoon. I get the corner room, the one I have been hoping for. But when I am left alone in it for the first time while the others are taught how to wash and gown and mask in the anteroom, it is very lonely and intimidating. I feel lost and immediately decide I want to go home. Just like in labor when you change your mind and decide you really don't want to have a baby after all.

But I stay, as Mark moves in my stereo, word processor and favorite artwork, which is not easy wearing a mask and gown. Peter helps by riding the bike. I am emotional and tearful but tell Mark to go home, get something to eat, and get a good night's sleep. He does and I cry as he walks out the door.

Can't sleep at all, listening to Sarah McLachlan on my earphones. I am completely convinced by now that she wrote the *Fumbling Towards Ecstasy* album for me and what I am going through and I cling to each word, each thought, each image. Every single night as I try to fall asleep, Sarah sings her strange lullabies to me.

Nurse Debi visits for a while. We have a good talk about my sexual abuse history and what I am hoping to accomplish with the stem cell rescue. At age 35, she discovers that she is adopted. When confronted, her parents are angry at her for being so disruptive and such a troublemaker. We have both dared to tell the family secret. And her father will not stand up for her with her mother. Just like my mother won't for us. We talk about how tired we are at age 37 and 42. We become instant friends. She has to get back to work. I reluctantly ask for a painkiller for the surgery discomfort at around 330 am, call Mark at 4 (he says I can anytime) and then finally get a couple hours sleep. Awake at 645, I turn over and gasp at the stunning pink sunrise I can see from my bed outside the big picture window.

My next door neighbor, whom I will never see, is only seventeen years old. A high school athlete with bone cancer also undergoing a transplant. He has been hooked up for three weeks and is having a rough time. I fantasize that we will send secret written messages under the door just as the POWs in Vietnam did.

I play the classics on my stereo and everyone who comes in loves the music. One of the doctors makes an "entrance" at a particular crescendo, which seems to delight him.

People are buzzing about a sign that appears on my door. Since I am not allowed to even poke my head out of the room, I don't know what they are talking about. Seems that Mark has posted a set of rules for Trish's room. They read:

TRISH'S ROOM RULES

The following are ABSOLUTELY PROHIBITED:
Anyone with an attitude (doctors not excepted)
Mushrooms
Negative vibes
MISTAKES
Jehovah's Witnesses (Sorry…already read Watchtower)
Certain friends and family (to be named at a later date… see first list item above)
Any health care professional not willing to discuss and/or explain, upon request, each and   every procedure, medicine, order, etc., from alcohol swabs on up
Large needles
Rigid catheters
Anyone proclaiming the joys of high dose chemotherapy
Wig salespersons
Germs
Square dancers
Cab drivers (claiming someone from this room called needing ride to airport)
Cold hands
Flowers
Books written by Robert James Waller
Platitudes
Referring to emesis basin as "emesis basin." Accepted terminology is "puke pan"
Kyle from UBS (if he's carrying a waste basket)
Well-intentioned visitors with stories of other cancer patients whose cancers have nothing to do with Trish's
People who talk at movies

GENERAL:
Residents must remain on leash at all times
Angels check wings at Nurses Station 3C (all that dust, you know,
celestial or otherwise)
Smile
Duck

OPTIONAL (but recommended):
Addressing Trish as "Your Highness"

CHAPTER SEVENTY-ONE

Saturday the chemo drips begin. I am pre-medicated based on the dosage in the protocol manual which I inform them will be way too much but they ignore me. Sure enough before she even finishes pushing the medication into my port, I am frightfully dizzy, threatening to faint, and throwing up. Wonder what the regular medication will do to me! I stay dizzy for a few hours, extremely exhausted and sleep unnaturally most of the day.

Sunday, I talk them out of the pre-medication. But I am pretty nauseous as the chemo continues to drip. I have a huge rolling stand about seven feet high that I call Igor which holds four pumps and six IV bags full of chemo and various other concoctions. This stand accompanies me wherever I go as I am hooked up to it by four ports on two catheters, one in my arm and one in my chest. Yes, it's cumbersome. But on Wednesday, chemo will be over and I will get unhooked for the rest of the time and the pick line in my arm will come out. That will be a good day.

Planning a bath.

Writing a letter.

Dear Michael,

I got your phone message this morning. I loved how I could feel how cold it was from the way your voice sounded.

Your painting has now been hung on the wall over the stereo where I can see it perfectly from my bed. I'm in the darkest center now, shedding the old. Still a delicate balance. The light grey is next, one step closer. Then tiptoe through the white to get to the glorious pink.

Reader's Digest "Points to Ponder" said that February is a splendid time to tune out the world and hibernate a little. Also that character contributes to beauty. It fortifies a woman as her youth fades. A mode of conduct, a standard of courage, discipline, fortitude and integrity can do a great deal to make a woman beautiful.

I am having a strong sense of fighting through the final stages of my old life now. A lot of physical discomfort, time to contemplate and prepare to bury and let go. I'm going to emerge soon.

> *Hold on*
> *Hold on to yourself*
> *For this is gonna hurt like hell*
> *Hold on*
> *Hold on to yourself*
> *You know that only time can tell*
> *What is it in me that refuses to believe*
> *This isn't easier than the real thing*
> *Am I in heaven or*
> *Am I in hell*
> *At the crossroads I am standing*
> *So now you're sleeping peaceful*
> *I lie awake and pray*
> *That you'll be strong tomorrow*
> *And will see another day*
> *And we will praise it*
> *And love the light that brings a smile*
> *Across your face*
> *Hold on*
> *Hold on to yourself*
> *For this is gonna hurt like hell*
> **—Sarah McLachlan**

CHAPTER SEVENTY-TWO

Day Zero has arrived, meaning the high dose chemo has nearly knocked out my immune system leaving me with virtually "zero" cells of any kind, and the doctor has called my family in to be present for the infusion of my bag of pretty stem cells into my now lifeless, immune system-less, worn out, drugged out, sad little body. He declares it my new birthday, calls it cause for celebration, instructs me to wear the white christening dress with pearls and lace that Mark bought for me, and seems to be looking forward to it. I am fretting slightly over the car trip my frozen stem cells will make from the blood bank to the transplant unit. What, I ask, happens if there is an accident and my stem cells are lost or destroyed? I am sitting in a sterile room without even a hint of an immune system and no way to make a new one without the stem cells. They assure me that the frozen bags are contained in a large metal can, similar to a beer keg, to protect them in case of impact. I ask about the technique used to "defrost" my precious cells and bring them to just the right temperature. They say, with straight faces, that they run them under warm water in the sink in my room until they aren't frozen anymore. Very high tech.

For the first time, the heart monitor over my bed is turned on and I get hooked up to it. I can't imagine that my body won't welcome its own stem cells back with open arms but just knowing they are monitoring my heart gives me concern that something could go wrong. I try not to think of the fantastically dangerous implications of stem cells that won't take hold, or have been improperly frozen and are not viable, or mistakenly actually belong to someone else because the wrong bag was grabbed from the freezer shelf. I am at the point of no return now that all the high dose chemo induced killing has taken place within my body. I contemplate the new role of faith in my life.

As my counts have continued to bottom out each day, I have felt increasingly empty and flat and strange. One day I was laying with my head sideways on the pillow, consciously contemplating how easy it would be to just close my eyes and drift away permanently. Not like suicide or giving up, just a conscious decision to let go and stop fighting against my disease and all the things in my life that made me so tired and sad, knowing how much work would be involved in building a new immune system, cell by cell, and starting a brand new life. My landscapers use burlap sheets to gather and tie up grass clippings. I have been feeling like one of their burlap squares, with a pulse. Barely a pulse. Flat, one dimensional, and without content. A book with nothing written on the pages. Choosing to go through with it means I will have to, and get to, write every word on the new pages of my life.

The doctor is running the frozen bag under the warm water now. I watch him suck my beautiful, thawed stem cells out of the bag with a huge hypodermic needle. He comes to me and slowly pushes life into my catheter, my own life. The best part of my former self that I saved to make my new self. I can feel the cells begin to move through me. It is what I perceive to be as close as a person can come to sensing and feeling the creation of life, the potential of cells to become life. Immediately I feel fuller, not so dead inside. It is hope swimming around inside.

CHAPTER SEVENTY-THREE

February 24th

A week has passed since I came in this room and it has been hell. My counts were not bottomed out completely when I was infused and they continue to crash, even though it is hard to believe that physically I could sink any lower. It is too early for the stem cells to take hold. Way too sick to write. Sitting on my fresh bed now, just had a shower (delicious) after a fucking miserable night. The drugs to keep my stomach under control leave thick paste in my mouth and cause violent, disturbing dreams. I'm lonely. No one touching me. An alien. Have had only a few bites of food in the past four days, very weak. Listening to that Irish woman sing. She's helping me. Called Mark twice in the night but he does not understand my deepest need in this new life. He is managing things and care brilliantly but not me personally. I wish it could be different.

My dear friend, Kathy, gave me a beautiful small white polar bear, that she calls Butterfly Bear in honor of my transformation. I keep him close like a child would. At this moment I feel faint stirrings of my beautiful new life arriving, the suffering beginning to subside. Currently trying to throw up my breakfast. Sending it back down. I think I can keep it there.

Last night was my deepest black hole, I hope. I think I am feeling better.

February 25th

It is the middle of the night, 225 am, the second night this hour has vexed me. This one more manageable than the last. Body feels decent but mouth, lips, nose are a trial. Lips raw as an arctic expedition, nose bloody, inside of mouth tight, tender and ready to fully bloom into violent sores at any minute. Then there is the miserable art of eating. Have to take a drug prior to each time or I simply wretch everything. Even when I can partake, it is with no interest and far more trepidation for spitting it up one more time. The deep hiccups are always full and shady.

Pete came to visit and play cards with me. I puked practically right in his lap with no warning and felt awful about it. He didn't seem to care at all but I thought it was a shitty thing for a mother to do to her kid.

Mark arrived later and gave me another wonderful warm lotion rub.

My sister visited. It was magical and mystical, like we had been waiting all our lives. She brought homemade food and was loving, caring, and affectionate. I was getting sleepy only because I felt deeply relaxed with her, safe. She left me to sleep and dream sweetly like a carefree child. Like a baby.

February 26th

My transplant coordinator says I look like Day +10 instead of Day +3 (counting forward from day of infusion of my own stem cells). My God, what do the others look like? Can't imagine that. Diarrhea, sore mouth, raw lips, upset stomach, no hair. Sometimes I cry. I'm coming back.

February 27th, Day +4

God, am I dead yet? When Mark left last night, I wasn't tired and doing decent. At 2 am I was sobbing, so lonely, hurting so bad. My mouth, my God. And the bloody congestion in my throat which hurts so bad. I just wanted a human being so bad and when I called Mark and he started talking about asking for drugs I hung up on him. Then I cursed Michael for not being with me. There must be a reason for all of this now. Suddenly it was Andrew I wanted, just like when I was throwing up my hair into the toilet. Mark, totally unsure of what to do with me by this time, agreed to see if he was awake. I said to wake him up. I cried to Andrew that I needed to see him soon. He took me and the phone with him into the bathroom to pee. I settled down and hung up. Laying in the dark with earphones and Butterfly Bear, I listened and hurt and cried. I wanted to call my mom but knew I could not. Then Katie, Nazi night nurse, barged in right behind my beautiful, big Andrew and demanded to know why I hadn't called her if I needed someone. I said I didn't want her. She did vitals, IV antibiotic, cleaned the bathroom, weighed me, and drew blood. And then I got my Andrew. He was emotionally wrecked due to having spent the evening with his girlfriend who had slept with his best friend, breaking Andrew's heart. He still loves her so much. We all love and miss her so much. She is like a daughter to me. He gave me the wonderful opportunity, in the dead of night, to listen, to help, to be his mom instead of a cancer patient. God's gift he is.

February 28th
The music I'm listening to in here will be indelibly etched on my psyche along with this place.

> *I love the time*
> *And in between*
> *The calm inside me in the space*
> *Where I can breathe*
> *I believe there is a distance*
> *I have wandered to touch upon the years of*
> *Reaching out and reaching in*
> *Holding out*
> *Holding in*

I believe
This is heaven
To no one else but me
And I'll defend it as long as
I can be
Left here to linger in silence
If I choose to
Would you try to understand

Oh the quiet child
Awaits the day
When she can break free
The mold that clings like desperation

Mother
Can't you see I've got to
Live my life the way I feel is
Right for me
Might not be right for you but it's
Right for me
—Sarah McLachlan

My horoscope says:
"Life will intensify for Pisces this month with Mars (the action and energizing planet) in Pisces February 15 through March 24. Gentle exercise will provide stress relief and a wonderful source of energy. You have a calm center now because you have heavenly help assisting you. That invisible good fairy—the one you have sensed hovering over you since birth—is astrologically close at hand this month, ready to wave her magic wand and return you into the fray of life again."

Sometimes it's hard to believe as I endure this experience that it is leading to anything but the grave. I often feel I am lying on the edge of death waiting to be pulled back. The fear, of course, is that I won't come back.

February 29th

Still feel a lot of pain. My esophagus and mouth sores have kicked in and all hell is breaking loose. Can't swallow, very bloody nose (low platelets), white count still at .1 which is nothing. Will need both bloods today (whole blood and platelets). God.

March 1st

What a day. I got two units of red blood and platelets yesterday. Hooked up a lot. Feel better but very weak. Platelets are at 9, almost nonexistent. Middle of the night, battling with Nazi nurse Katie, nose went nuts. Bloody congestion. She turned up the humidity in the room and it was like a bloody faucet. It was so miserable for five hours. Throat and esophagus still raw down to tummy. I have to plan to swallow. It is excruciating. My christening gown is covered with blood. I am pretty rock bottom, so bloody and miserable. Doc says if platelet transfusions don't hold pretty soon we will have to seek out more genetically compatible donations, maybe my sister. But my platelet transfusion was remarkable this time. I literally sucked up the bag in seven minutes. Felt better right away. So they tracked down that particular angel donor, who must remain anonymous to me, and he made two additional donations. Nurse Patti got me through in her fabulous know-exactly-what-to-say-and-what-not- to-say way. She alone contributed to this most important day, pulled me through. I'm beginning to notice that the vast majority of those on my angel lists have RN next to their names. My white cells have made a move. .2!!! Finally I am moving in the right direction.

Had a brief but wonderful visit with Dr. John who had not been on hospital rotation since I had been admitted. Asked if I would appear on a local television segment with him about the clinic. He said he wanted someone articulate and someone he could control. He said he knew the latter was impossible with me. We laughed and I accepted with joy.

Lavender Regina, a small purplish teddy bear, arrived in a balloon package sent by a big client. She has joined Butterfly Bear to help take care of me. She is a bit of a snob but then so am I.

Enjoying the few evenings where Mark leaves a little earlier and I have some quiet time to myself. Michael called last night after I had snoozed off. It almost seems like a dream now.

When Dr. John was in, I mentioned how unpleasant all the chemo side effects were. His comment was "Yeah, but just think how we eradicated those cancer cells. I'll bet there is not one left in your body. We won!" His eyes glistened and gleamed behind the mask.

March 2nd, 5:45 am
I triumphantly slept through the night! Kept my platelets, I'll bet. Counts are up, I'll bet. Had to push hard at the dreaded 2 am evil time but did mouth care (seriously painful) and asked Debi for Tylenol and struggled on through. What joy. Just like a baby. Slept through the goddamned night!!

My job now is to make cells and I do it like crazy. Deep into the night, my feet burn and I feel as if my bones are working out. This activity signals new cells and I become familiar and comfortable with the feeling. I don't want to move when it is happening, creating a perfect stillness in which the internal work takes place. It is the advanced version of the initial feeling of the stem cells being pushed into my veins. First they swam around and now they are established, busy, busy at work, multiplying and creating a community of life within me. I will never forget this feeling. I will never forget how I made every cell in my body all by myself from scratch in the middle of the night in a sterile room. I cannot wait for 530 am to come. I am wide awake and know that the blood they will draw from my catheter will prove how much work I have done overnight. Sometimes the cells double in number. I am really good at this.

March 3rd, 5:45 am

Yesterday was full of highs and lows. Count went from .2 to .5!! Platelets holding. I felt great. Had a super energized morning. Of course, got my butt kicked by nausea at lunchtime, puked up some, got sick off the IV antibiotic with diarrhea. Then got very unpleasant when on late rounds a suggestion was made that I should get out of bed and work out more. Mark left early at 630 pm. Hard for us both but it was the right thing. I was totally exhausted by 8 but suddenly realized that I didn't feel safe sleeping at 8, not keeping watch. Forced myself to confront the fear, turned out the light and slept. Woke up around 10 and had a great talk with Mark about it. How I can be safe now. Debi hunted me down a strawberry popsicle in the middle of the night which was a revelation. First time the pain of swallowing seemed reduced. Slept well after that, feeling more normal in my body. I've almost made it through. Debi sat with me for an hour around 5 am. It was such an unexpected pleasure. She is a loving caring person with a broken heart. Told me about Jillian, the nurse in her thirties who ten years ago had ovarian cancer, was having (and hating) chemo, thought it was killing her. Her three year old died (drowned) in the back yard while she was in the hospital. Her husband later killed himself. She quit chemo and cured herself. Ten years out now, remarried to a hunk. She also has long beautiful red hair.

Looking out my window, I can see the beginnings of another spectacular sunrise. I look onto the McDowell Mountain range which frames the changing colors. I crank my bed way up off the floor and sit transfixed for thirty minutes until regrettably the usual blue/grey morning sky appears and the day begins. The air-brushed clouds reflect the brilliant pinks with the mountains looking like dark jewels behind. The transformation has truly occurred for me now and everything does feel different.

All that I hoped for and more.
All the fear has left me now
I'm not frightened anymore
It's my heart that pounds beneath my flesh
It's my mouth that pushes out this breath
And if I shed a tear I won't cage it
I won't fear love
And if I feel a rage I won't deny it
I won't fear love

Peace in the struggle to find peace
Comfort on the way to comfort
—Sarah McLachlan

It is Sunday. I will have good counts again. I will leave my room to walk to x-ray tonight. I will be released next week.

CHAPTER SEVENTY-FOUR

I write letters on this Monday, beginning to feel myself moving towards the close of my time in the hospital.

March 4th

Dear Michael,

I've reread your letter many times. I certainly entered this place with a strong desire to have you with me. But this has become an increasing problem for me. Unlike you, I cannot harbor that kind of desire and need and manage it in a positive way. It permeates my inner life and seeps into my outer life and makes it impossible to find the peace I've been seeking. This being very ironic because you have brought me more peace in my life than I have ever known. I'm hoping that with my new life, I can get close to your sister's perspective and accept you as the gift you are to me. Without needing and wanting it to be more. I am no longer afraid of your love. I want it, relish it, rely on it, and revel in it. But it was good that you couldn't be here. Healthier for both of us, forcing me to buck up on my own. I fully admit that the incredible glimpse of closeness, trust, unconditional love, and deep spiritual connection that you have introduced me to has put me into something of a spin. But I want to make sure our feelings are not tainted by guilt, secrecy, and constant pain. The feelings are too pure and perfect for that.

I reread my own letter. I feel the change in my words. The move towards bringing my life into focus. The transformation.

To: Dr. Bernie Siegel author of *Love, Medicine and Miracles*

I feel that I have experienced my own birth. I have seen my beautiful stem cells come out of my body and two months later go back in to do their work for me. Which they have done brilliantly as I knew they would. I have had the trauma and pain and humiliation and shame and suffering killed off with my old bone marrow and I have been reborn. To be honest, I think I could have kicked the cancer without the rescue, but I wouldn't have missed it for the world. I cared enough about myself to risk everything to have myself back. I brought pictures of me as a child to put on my special bulletin board in the hospital because recapturing that child and her joy and innocence was the goal. Every new hair I had grown has now fallen out again from the high dose chemo. And I look amazingly like the beautiful bald baby in the picture again. I feel like a newborn as well. Full of joy, hope and promise. In this amazing process, I have also felt love come towards me that I could never allow before. And I have been able to love in a new and very profound way. The incredible kindness and concern of those who have cared about me has been a revelation. God has answered every one of my prayers. He gave me cancer. I know you understand that. I am quite certain that my body will never host cancer again. I do not live in fear but instead, as you taught me, treasure every moment of every beautiful day of my new life no matter what its length may be. I find myself sometimes feeling sorry for people who will never get this wonderful opportunity. I happily and gratefully take your spirit into my new life with me.

To my nutritionist and his wife:

Dear Richard and Kathy,

As you know, I have been astounding medical science with my progress the past two days. The first mention of nutrition by the esteemed medical team came as my body began this remarkable recovery from the dead. The doctor deadpans that my potassium is on the low side of normal so let's start taking these horse pills after meals when they are more easily tolerated. I am, of course, suspicious so I call Richard and ask for the real scoop. He curses lightheartedly, something about how he really doesn't like to get into these things but since I pick up on everything, yes, the horse pill does irritate the intestines. (Oh, great, I'm thinking, just what I need. A new irritation of the intestines.) Richard reluctantly and modestly admits, with prodding, that his Mineral Replacement product would be better. I tell Mark to bring it from home but it doesn't happen until the following morning. Meanwhile, I hide the horse pills. I am told with raised eyebrows by the team that morning that the potassium is not going up so now we are going to double the horse pills. (And double the irritation, no doubt.) I smile again and accept the pills from the team, hiding them in my special lemon drop tin. Mark arrives with the goods and gently admonishes me for not being honest with the team. I begin popping Mineral Replacement with lots of water for the rest of the day, just praying I won't get caught. With meals, in between meals, and in the night. Always on the sly. (I think my nurse suspects.) I go to sleep with difficulty due to all the excitement of the day, going from .5 to 2.6 white cells overnight. Astounding, says the team. I know I am building more cells because the bottom of my feet are burning and I am sweating a bit. Still haven't spiked that fever they promised I would, never got into triple digits one time. I wake up at 2 am, with a strange but oddly familiar sensation. The urge to pee. The whole time I have been here, the team has been saying that I don't pee enough while I'm wondering when the pee stops being so thick and disgusting. So I go to my bathroom and, for the first time in over two weeks, have a normal, thin stream of clear urine. Then, in another bold move, the first normal bowel movement as well. Not diarrhea and not painful. Felt like a plain old-fashioned "dump," as my boys would say. I have this huge smile on my face knowing, of course, that the Mineral Replacement is doing much more than I asked of it. When I got up and admired my work, I dabbed the sore spots with your vital-E lotion I keep in the bathroom, popped a couple more illicit Mineral Replacements, and called the nurse to clean up the mess (well, they insist on seeing and measuring everything). Would you believe she did not even compliment me on the nice pee and the pretty dump? After all that bitching. Now I know it is time to go home from the hospital and get well. Seriously, folks, this is a true story and perhaps can only be fully appreciated by me and Butterfly Bear and our new friend Regina but my hope is that you will understand the value of what you have spent a career doing and caring about. Call me arrogant, but if it only saved me, I think it was worth it, you know. And it has saved me. No chance my little body could have withstood the rigors of this ordeal without you and I would have never had the confidence to try. I will not forget and I will not be quiet. And will never stop thanking you.

CHAPTER SEVENTY-FIVE

March 5th

Dear Michael,
The doctors played a little joke on me this morning and came in for
rounds without their masks on. I shrieked and pulled the sheet over my
mouth and demanded to know where their masks were. They laughed,
eyes sparkling, and said they didn't need their masks anymore. I'm
sprung and was complimented on a great "performance." I am sitting
at my little desk looking out the big picture window to the mountains.
Cars are driving by, the park is green, and I will soon be part of it.
It's cloudy but every now and then the sun bursts out right onto my
face. I'm feeling totally ready to leave now and got a great Trish rush
when I pulled on my jeans for the first time in eighteen days. It's all
starting to come back. I want to go to the movies, I want to dance, to
write and to smile and laugh and love my kids.

I'm going home.

March 6th

I woke up at 430 am in anticipation of my 530 blood test that I knew
was going to send me home officially. I watched the sunrise for the
last time out my big window to the world. And before 7, I took my
now allowed walk through the halls, mask on, of course. That was
an interesting experience. Not only did I discover that the nurses
are a chatty little bunch, mostly talking about us patients, but that

the oncology floor of a major hospital is a pretty desperate place and I fought a case of survivor's guilt.

I began packing, an emotional experience. The things that had formed my world for those incredible eighteen days were now being broken down and my new life, that I fought so hard to have, was about to be implemented. The nurse stuck her head in and I could tell by her smile and enthusiasm that my blood test was good enough. She said it looked like I was going home. The doctor arrived on rounds. He is not a real dynamic guy and does not know what to make of me. But his idea of a joke was to bring in the menus for the following day, like I would be needing them. I threw them in the trash can and proclaimed I would take my meals at home from now on. He smiled and confirmed.

The boys (all three) arrive and start loading up. Mark very sensitively takes loads with one son at a time, leaving the other to stay with me. It doesn't take long and we are ready to go. Suddenly, I am overwhelmed with emotion and begin to cry. I ask them all to wait for me outside with the obligatory wheelchair so that I may say my private good-byes to the room that almost killed me and certainly saved me, the room where I didn't want to stay on the first night and now can barely bring myself to leave. As a final gesture, I erase the greaseboard that has marked my progress and the number of days I have been here and also has the funny drawings the boys did for me. I just can't leave it blank so I write a message to the next occupant, offering good luck and encouragement. Then I walk out of my room, the most difficult and grandest exit of my career.

Mark had my beautiful car detailed that very morning, laughing that he almost scheduled it too late because I got out so unexpectedly early. My Mayo team tells me that I have broken the record for the fastest in and out of a stem cell rescue or transplant of any kind.

CHAPTER SEVENTY-SIX

The house is perfectly clean, organized and spotless under my mother's supervision the last few days. I have fantasized over this possibility for years so I guess we can just chalk it up to another blessing of cancer. There are new sheets and blankets on all beds, towels, and all kinds of other surprises. It is glorious.

Mark goes off to the store to get prescriptions filled and the boys and I spend the most wonderful hour or so in my room, laughing and enjoying each other so much. No direct mention of the incredible relief of my return, but it's in the air. Peter stays very close all day and finally leaves me after I drift off for a quick nap from total exhaustion. Later I help him with his state capitals for a test, snuggle up in my chair with my blanket, have dinner and go to sleep in my own bed.

March 9th

Wasn't feeling so well yesterday and having been well trained from the clinic to keep an eye on fevers, asked Andrew to get the thermometer. After having been the only patient they ever had that did not run a fever during the entire transplant, I was shocked and horrified to see that the thermometer read 101.3. I gasped and called the clinic immediately. They insisted I come down right away. I don't think I had been that scared through this entire ordeal. I had done so well and my head was immediately filled with visions of not being able to fight this thing off, or it being pneumonia or some other ghastly thing. I could just see the concern on their faces when I arrived at the clinic. They took a ton of blood (after having optimistically removed the catheter just the day before) and I had to get stuck twice which was something I have not missed with the luxury of the catheter. Was given antibiotics and strict instructions while we waited for the blood cultures to come back after the weekend. Fever went down shortly after I got home and I got extra sleep and was able to eat. Just a virus and, by God, I fought it off rather nicely. Quite a scare, though.

March 14th

I am really enjoying the rain this morning. Both boys are sleeping in. I make homemade coffee cake which is in the oven, and sleep in til 8 am. I have been getting up real early and going to the studio to work out. But this morning I am just enjoying hanging out and taking it easy. Besides, my muscles are so sore from trying to find their way back that they can probably use a little break. It is a good hurt though, better than the chemo kind, the needle kind, or the bone marrow biopsy kind. Weighed in at a little over 105 yesterday and rising fast.

Today I feel ready to start my recovery collage. Don't know why I had to wait but it is still such a tender spot. I weep as I sort through the things I want to preserve. I feel so cherished and treasured now. Finally. I am saved.

March 16th

My last day of being 42. What will always be known to me as my cancer year. Whew. I slept so much better last night. More myself. Must have been finishing the mega-antibiotics I've been on. I'm still in bed, listening to Irish music and writing little notes to friends. Mark is taking me to Vincent's tonight, late at 915 so it won't be too crowded. He says that I have earned this birthday with my own blood, sweat and tears. (I guess I did not know the meaning of that phrase until now.) He loves me. I'm happy. I'm pretty well. I'm certainly okay. So I have had to work a little harder than most to have a life to look forward to. And I love every little minute of it.

March 17th, St. Patrick's Day, my birthday

We slept in a bit this morning and Mark went to get us croissants, all of our favorite kinds. So all of us got to get up and eat ours whenever we pleased. The boys took me to a movie in the afternoon. I wasn't feeling so great when we got home so laid down in my room until Mark had the birthday dinner ready.

Didn't feel too great yesterday either. Stayed in bed most of the day and didn't feel well enough to get up and go to the studio until around 630 in the evening. Perked up pretty good then and actually had the energy to dance for a while after the warm-up which I have not had the stamina to do. Also having some pretty good aching in my knees and long bones, which I assume is a result of all the exercise and the still very active bone marrow. I am learning the art of napping and resting and slowing down which I am sure will be a valuable lesson. It sure feels strange though.

Right now I am so tender emotionally, trying to adjust to all these new feelings I am experiencing. I feel a tremendous amount of joy and peace and contentment, more than I ever thought possible. And that is how I have healed myself. I am enjoying this quiet time with my family as this illness has presented an opportunity for a lot of healing for us as a family. There is still a delicate balance for me between the physical frailty, the emotional renewal, and dealing with the strain of it all.

I have noticed in the past two days, even though I have not felt particularly well, that my face is beginning to look healthy again. My skin, my color, a bit of healthy glow returning. I looked at myself for quite a while this afternoon and felt, for the first time, that I could see my recovery happening. Life is beginning to breathe back into my system, my brand new system.

March 20th

Vincent's was rough. Very crowded, which made me nervous. The hostess tells us that our waiter's sister just had the same "surgery" as me. To my horror, he sits down at the table with us after dinner and tells every detail of his sibling's bone marrow transplant. Tough way to spend our big evening out. Kind of a bust.

I woke up at 2 am with nightmares about too many people too close to me. But I'm okay. This whole at home recovery period has no real definition or boundary. I kind of float through each day. I try to nap, listen to music, be calm. We go to movies when no one else does and I spend short periods of time at the office after the others go home.

I'm feeling pretty well except for the bone and joint pain. I talked to someone at the clinic who thought it was overtraining but mentioned x-rays to look for bone involvement. I took this pretty hard, the fear factor, but nutritionist and Mark talked me down. Nothing points to that. I've laid off the last two days and it doesn't hurt so bad. People still amaze me with their concern, gestures, and generous spirit. Flowers, cards, books, tapes, prayers. I feel so loved and cherished and have missed that so in my previous life. I'm sure I have been healed with help from another power. I've been held in some loving arms.

Things are good at home. Boys are back to normal.

Mark and I quietly proceeding. Close and involved. The first time we talked about sex, I said that with my transformation came a new attitude and I wasn't sure how I felt. He lay close by and said I could decide when I was ready and for what. By the time we were through talking, we were well on our way to our first intimacy in my new life. It worked beautifully. Unlike what I was told to expect, my body knew what to do and did well. I was happy and relieved. Things have been okay since.

There is a part of me, private and deep, that still exists elsewhere in a safe and wonderful place. Don't know its spot in my life yet. Patience. Deep breaths, living in the moment, accepting and not trying to control.

In the bath now. Mark promises one of his special hot lotion rubs when I'm out. And so it wonderfully goes. . .

CHAPTER SEVENTY-SEVEN

I begin to feel the aftershock of the audacity of my decision to keep my parents away from me. Now that I am out of the hospital, they are beginning to bristle. My sister tells me that they did not disclose to their friends and extended family that they were not welcome in my transplant room, using whatever second hand information they were hearing and my occasional update faxes to further their image of a happy, close family in peril. Peter is still livid with them over an incident that occurred while I was hospitalized. They asked him to come over to pick up some food my mother had made for me. We knew that my father had been ill so Peter was instructed to stay at the front door, take the food, and have no contact with either of them to insure that he did not bring the illness back to my sterile room. When he arrived, they assured him that Papa was not really sick and he should come in the house. He refused, not willing to risk it. But they teased him about it, insisted he come in, put their hands on him, and completely ignored his pleas to be cautious for my benefit. He was scared to death that I would catch whatever his grandfather had. We later learned that my father's lab work came back positive, meaning he really was sick and contagious when Peter was at their home picking up the food. And my mother is none too pleased that she worked hard cleaning up my house for my return but still isn't welcome to visit during this very early tender phase of my

post-transplant recovery. At one point, she suggests that I would
be better off recuperating at their home. The very thought of it is
terrifying. I express my feelings in a letter.

March 24th

Dear Mom,

*So I hear that you are pretty angry at me for not giving you what you
want. WOW!!! I thought cancer (high risk life-threatening variety)
gave me special privileges. Like deciding what would be the most
advantageous environment in which to attempt a transplant, or in
which to recuperate quietly and without risk. Guess not. I should
have remembered from your careful teachings when I was a child to
put your needs first. Let you invade my hospital room at your will
and then recuperate at your house because it is "cleaner." But since I
didn't go along with that, you decided to attempt to clean my house,
which admittedly was a huge task. Guess I didn't understand the
rule that if you clean my house, you get to come over whenever you
want. And I thought you just cleaned it as a loving parental gesture.
Helping out, you know. Silly me. God, I seem so confused.*

*So about all of my supporters which you cultivate and manage so
well. It must be hell to try to keep them properly informed in your role
as keeper of Trish when Trish isn't cooperating at all. How do you tell
them what my hospital room looks like or how I am looking? Do you
make it up? Or do you just say that there is a horrible secret history
of sexual abuse in our family and Trish just got tired of living in that
black hole so she decided not to bring that shit into her brand new
life of her own creation? So you don't really know how I look or how
I am doing. Except for my faxes that Kathy says you love so well. I
couldn't understand how you could be so angry but loved to get those
faxes. Well, she explained that it gives you the necessary information
to keep those lies going.*

*And then there is this business about Kathy being so loving and
cooperative with you when she is the only obvious victim of the big*

secret. And, of course, nothing really happened to me so what the hell do I think I am dong? If the big victim can come around, I certainly have no right to rock the boat so viciously. Isn't that irritating? Don't you hate it when that happens? I guess Kathy just seems to remember her early childhood and adolescent training a lot better than I do.

Well, you always have the boys, right? Ummm, maybe not. Peter is pretty pissed about that day when Dad had the virus and you assured him that he didn't. You insisted that Peter come in the house and have physical contact with his grandfather even though he very much wished to stay at the door as I had instructed him carefully to do. (He obviously does not understand the part about the victims giving up all their rights to the abusers.) I guess you didn't realize how tough it must have been for Pete to come to the hospital wondering if he brought that virus with him. And then finding out that the lab work was indeed positive. And then you both doing that thing you do when you have really gone too far and you know it. You each called me individually to say that you didn't really do what Peter reported you had. Mom, you said that you handed him the food with gloves on. And Dad, you said you didn't get near him. This really pissed Peter off. Now the two adults question the veracity of the statement of the child to cover their asses. Good technique. Hated to see Peter served up on the silver platter like that. I thought that was a privilege reserved for me and my sister. I guess not.

Later, a few days after I had come home from the hospital, Peter gave me some advice. He said that you two were the most likely to attempt to take my beautiful new life, for which I worked so hard, and yank it back to the old toxic ways. He said not only did he support my not seeing you or talking to you, he insisted on it. What could I say?

You know, sometimes I get weak and emotional and think that I should just call you and come to visit. This actually happens quite often. And just when I am about to do so, you do something that absolutely validates my present course of action. For that I thank you.

I don't actually send the letter to my parents. Instead I just continue sending the regular faxes with updates on how I am doing. My thinking is that I no longer want to engage in difficult discussions with them that are bound to be upsetting with no possibility of success. So I just write what I would say if they could actually listen and feel better once it is out of me. I am beginning to see how very inconvenient this situation is for my parents, how threatening it is to their cover-up and denial. It is clear to me that while they will never admit it, or even consciously consider it, it would be easier for them if cancer just killed me. Then they could mourn the tragic loss of their daughter for all to see and live in the martyrdom of their grief for all time. Instead, I pull off this miraculous recovery which doesn't include them and there is no plausible explanation for our estrangement at a time when one would normally expect a family to be very close. Except the truth, of course. Since that is not an option, I continue to be a difficult impediment to their carefully constructed image. I have a vision of being laid out dead on a silver platter, served up for the last time, the ultimate sacrifice of a daughter to meet the needs of her parents.

March 25th, Day +31

Difficult weekend. Very tough, long talk with my sister. Since my immediate disease is no longer holding the family together, things are beginning to crumble and abuse issues take their hold once again. So much pain. Mark did his "I'm out of commission sexually" speech which clobbered me real good. I freaked out in all the worst ways. Trying to hang on. I subjected Mark to three hours of discussion regarding all of this mess. He has issues, too, not just me. He has to work so hard to love me. I can't stand that. He's angry and hostile in some ways. I'm sure that now that I am out of immediate danger, he feels he can begin to express his own emotions about reading my journal and dealing with my "affairs." He has an answer for all this. We agreed that I would get a place in Coronado at the beach in June to have that time alone. For both of us to have some time. I love the idea. I will probably have radiation between now and then. Then it is really over. Then I will grow hair. Then I get to go. I'm struggling here. God, this is hard.

CHAPTER SEVENTY-EIGHT

March 26th, Day +30

Check-up goes real well. Great numbers. They pitch follow-up radiation. My pains are rheumatism syndrome, post-chemo, which can last up to six months. Trying to cultivate my independence. . .with Mark. He's in that phase. Can't dwell on it. Working on my collage.

A Vision. . .

I'm standing on the Navy Seal training beach in Coronado wearing only my favorite sweatshirt. No hair anywhere. The Navy Seal, tall and thin, that I have seen practicing flowing Chinese exercises, approaches me from behind and I sense his presence, his mission. He turns me to face him and envelops me with his energy. He kisses me deeply, constantly. He fills me inside with himself. Soon he is sending a silver radiating matter all through me, lighting me up inside, traveling through my body. He urges me to let go and fully accept this healing gift, which I do. He then picks me up and carries me into the ocean. At waist deep, he whistles and the dolphins arrive. One is old, large, gentle and approaches and beckons me. The Seal places me on the back of the huge, friendly animal, chest down. I am no longer wearing my sweatshirt. I'm nude. The dolphin gently rides me through the water knowing exactly when to allow me air. I seem to be able to breathe freely. The vision never ends. It becomes my new life.

March 29th

Woe is me. I'm living in blah land, not here nor there. Radiation has reared its ugly head. Recurrence—survival-odds—percentages— blah, blah, blah. Depressed, lethargic. Face is tight or is it numb? I worry about everything. Thought I would put off the treatment for a week and go to Washington and New York for cherry blossoms, daffodils, dear friends. Can't find a decent fare. Mark is upset. I'm freaking out. Feel like I'm trapped—in my disease, in my house. HELP! Want to go to sleep. Want to run away. Want health. . .wind. . .stamina. . . love. . .affection. . .kindness. . .art. . .peace. Butterfly Bear is my friend. We're working on Miss Regina.

Next morning. . .

I have slept on it. I'm not going East. I'm taking Mark to Coronado. Only one night. Dinner at Prima Vera. Look at my June condo. I made reservations in our married name. This is right. He has endured the trauma with me the whole time and has the same needs of escape. I can't go to Michael after seeing the pain it causes Mark. Besides, going to Michael may just cause more pain. I feel uplifted by the rightness of this. Today I will shop, work on the collage, dance and we're eating out. I will show my husband love and respect. Just plain love.

April 2nd

Taped the television interview for the Mayo piece today at the dance studio. Of course, pushed too hard on the dance segments so I am already sore. I knew the cameraman from other projects and he was so dear, animated, friendly and loving. The producer was sensitive and emotional about my story. I had a wonderful time, so at ease with this process.
Ran into a woman in the grocery store who approached me because I was wearing a scarf so she spotted me for chemo. She had metastatic breast cancer, diagnosed during her seventh pregnancy. She was

tough but sad, talking transplant but probably out of the question in her case. She's had three years of chemo. A great need to convince me she could survive. I am often approached by people who need to share their stories. I listen and cry inside.

My friend, Frankie, the geologist, told me how emeralds undergo a type of radiation to bring out their most brilliant color and texture. He said I should think of radiation in the same way for myself. I adopt that image and decide it will be one of my major visualizations during the seemingly countless radiation treatments. A beautiful, brilliant emerald when it is all over.

April 5th

Just arrived back from Coronado where I proudly leased #508, El Camino tower, right on the beach, for the month of June. Gorgeous day today, breezy and cool yesterday. Two very long walks to my usual spot, where I spoke with God, thanking him for allowing me back to Coronado, which I begged for the week before my transplant, standing in exactly the same spot. I renewed my promise to give back in exchange for being saved, also acknowledging how brilliantly orchestrated my saving was by Him. Still have some weak spots, still working on that. Need so much love right now.

The moon led us back to our room from Prima Vera by foot. We left the door wide open to the ocean and snuggled in the soft bed with the luxurious sheets. I awoke at 230 am with the brilliant full moon casting fresh moonlight all across our bed. It was breathtaking and I just wanted to stay awake. 6 am. . .bright sunshine, no breeze and a cloudless blue sky. Glorious! Great breakfast on the balcony. Mark was sweet and flexible. No TV, great sex. . .so good.

Easter Sunday, April 7th

It has been a very nice day. Snuggles and sex in the morning, a work-out, breakfast with everyone, a movie, and cooking a big Easter dinner. I made banana cream pie. Listened to Ray Charles in the kitchen and was successfully able to move through the strong sense of my father in that music (his favorite). Then I just enjoyed it, pure and simple. An amazing accomplishment. Nice dinner, me and my boys. My mother-in-law told me on the phone to "eat a lot and do what you want." I loved her for that. If she only knew! I feel free and pure and clean and happy and uncontrolled and uncontrolling.

Tomorrow I will start my radiation treatments. I really struggled in the decision to go ahead but Peter convinced me with his seemingly urgent need for me to agree. He said he would take me every single day if I wanted him to. (I suspected it was just an excuse to miss a lot of school.) He is afraid I will not get enough treatment. Wants me to have it all. So I will find a way to be brave yet one more time. Thank God Mark is always there with me, holding my hand, and giving me the confidence to continue. I am glad I got to see my little beach condo so that every time I climb up on that metal table, I will close my eyes and imagine myself free as a bird, looking out over the ocean, smelling the salty air, finished with treatment, and moving completely into my new life. I can do it!!!

April 8th

Dear Michael,

And on my very first day, no radiation, just a set-up. Still I had to do quite a bit of visualizing to get through it. This is very hard, very hard for me. I can't shake the feeling that the transplant gave me all the healing I need and I shouldn't be subjecting myself to this radiation every day for six weeks. But it seems to mean so much to Peter that I can't bring myself to refuse. I mean, what if I didn't do enough when he told me to do more?

We should be languishing about writing long letters with feather plumes, not talking about radiation.

April 10th

I'm three days into the radiation process. My right arm is stiff and sore, I assume because I was hitched up in an awkward position for 25 minutes on Monday in simulation. I feel heavy tonight. Old like before, slipping back somehow. I wish I could visit with Michael. In person. Feel his lightness, his spirit, his feelings. To lift me up. Relieve the heaviness. Wish I could.

April 13th

I have been blue a bit, feeling depressed and fat. I'm really in good shape (did seven minutes stair master and fifteen minutes bike this morning) but the daily radiation is a mental test. So far no real side effects but a very sore right arm from all the tugging for position.

April 15th

I told Mark when I came home that I was free. At least a bit freer than yesterday. This came about as a result of a long conversation with Michael this afternoon in which I never felt weak or frustrated or unhappy or achy. Instead I just enjoyed the contact in a very healthy way.. I do not need him for my happiness. I look to myself more now. Takes pressure off Mark also. No anger and resentment like before. I can see more clearly the reality of it all in focus. That has been difficult up until now in my heightened state of emotion and cosmic "life and death" awareness. And Michael has been a brilliant reflection. Very gifted. I love him very much. But we will never be together. For the same reasons we couldn't be when I was 16 years old and I let him drive away from Myrtle Beach.

Had a wonderful massage. When I had the tumor inside of me, massage made me very ill. Now it is refreshing and uplifting.

April 20th

Radiation is getting a bit more intrusive. Friday's treatment made me real sleepy in the car, unnaturally so. And dark fatigue for a while when I get home. Work through it. Still no burn, just tightness mostly. Under arm area is better. Four weeks to go.

Hair sprouting everywhere. It's an amazing thing to experience. Like springtime in my body.

Sex is so much sweeter now for me. All cleaned up, you know. And very nice with Mark lately. He seems to be able to be more gentle and caring and vulnerable, probably because I'm not a barracuda anymore. His hands especially, stroking and lightly exploring. It's divine. I'm very happy. A new person but still trying to learn how.

April 21st

I feel safe, contented, cared for, happy and loved in Mark's arms. He has found a way to express himself, physically and emotionally like never before. Last night, having a drink at our favorite restaurant, I just laid my head on his shoulder and he was right there, accepting and protecting. Earlier, during dinner, I put my feet between his legs and he rubbed my bare feet throughout the evening. Then I choked on my big antibiotic pill and he was calmly ready for the Heimlich maneuver. To save me. Perhaps he has saved me. From a lot of things.

Bad dream. Waiting in large waiting room of doctor's office with two new young children and Mark. In walks my sister and my mother wearing ridiculous, cheap wigs on top of their heads. Then my father. They all say that Mark has arranged for them to take the kids for the weekend. I panic and say to Mark that we are just repeating mistakes and he turns into my father right in front of my eyes! Real bad.

Hair is growing.. Dark and soft. Between my legs, too.

April 22nd

Peter took me to radiation treatment this morning for the second time. He was interested in seeing the treatment room, the big radiation machine, and how it all works. So my very nice technicians gave him the tour and then let him sit in the computer control room and see how they control the radiation. He said repeatedly how much better he felt after seeing everything and how impressive the computer set-up was so that it seemed almost impossible for anything to really go wrong. He was also impressed by the huge door that automatically shuts before the radiation begins (with the big, intimidating radiation symbol on the door which always reminds me of a scary movie). They, of course, are all safely outside the door and I am the only poor soul inside with the machine. Sometimes it is too scary to think about. I get approximately one hundred times the exposure of an x-ray every day. God. Today I finished the second week with four to go. One third of the way through. Unfortunately, it gets a little more difficult as it continues because it has a cumulative effect. The tech calls it radiation fatigue and with some people it is constant and sometimes episodic. I overcome the feeling usually within a few hours of the treatment but it is pretty unpleasant. So far I have avoided any burning of the skin.

Mark brought some pictures back from the developers yesterday and they were sitting on the desk when I got home so I just grabbed them to take a look. I have absolutely no recollection of him taking them but there were several in the hospital during the transplant especially during the first few days of high dose chemo. I was so shocked when I saw those pictures, at the way I looked, at how much I cannot remember (thank God), at the magnitude of what happened to me there, I was overwhelmed with emotion. I had already forgotten the true physical misery and its profound effect on me. Even some photos he took about twelve days after I got home still looked pretty rough. It is so much for me to digest. The radiation has been a big hurdle for me to overcome and I am just barely able to conjure up the energy and positive spirit to go there every day and participate properly. I feel that it is going to be very close during the next four weeks, particularly as the fatigue and dosage continues to escalate. It is really rough on me. I am just flat running out of emotional steam. I hold a beautiful seashell in my hands during each treatment that Mark picked up for me in Coronado as we prepared to start this. I just try to visualize that on May 20th, I will be finished and on June 1st I will be at my little condo on the ocean. Honestly, I am in tears at this very moment just thinking of all this. I have truly just about reached my limit.

April 24th

Dear Peter,

I tried to call you when I got out of my treatment but you had already left for school. I knew that you would be so proud of me that I couldn't wait to tell you so I am leaving this note in your car. (I have already used the word "I" too many times, haven't I?)

I got up the nerve to wear my baseball cap into the clinic this morning, knowing this was the day that it was right to show my almost hairless head. And I was right, too. (Besides when I wear the baseball hat you let me borrow into the radiation room, it is sort of like having you in there with me. And, after all, radiation was kind of your idea, wasn't it?) Anyway, when I came out, I saw this young man who had been brought on a bed in an ambulance from the transplant unit to have his radiation. He was, of course, wearing a mask, waiting for his turn after me. I went up to him and the nurse who was with him and introduced myself, asking if he was from transplant. They said, yes, so I told him I was out of the hospital seven weeks yesterday. We both had on our baseball hats, Pete, so it was kind of like letting him know for sure that we had been going through the same thing. He is going to be transplanted tomorrow after two radiation treatments today. He was in pretty good spirits and I promised him there would be an end to all of this treatment, that I was three and a half weeks away from being finished. He smiled and seemed encouraged by seeing me so well and happy. I had a good cry after that, feeling so much for that guy and what he is going through. When I left, one of the ambulance drivers stopped me and said how cool it was that I shared that with him.

Anyway, I wanted to let you know how much you have influenced me in all of this. Your insistence on the radiation is what gave me the courage to keep going when I was ready to quit and be done. But it was the right thing to do. And thanks for taking me and caring about what happens to me when I am there. Through all of this, you have been such a great motivation for me to beat this and come out the other side so I can be your mom for as long as you want and need me. I love you.

April 25th

Just images today. Bad karma. Had to wait excessively for blood test, which ruined my concentration for radiation. New shields so time is longer on second and third angle. Mrs. White's Golden Rule Café ran out of chicken. Rusty Pelican ran out of mahi mahi. All I seem to do is get radiated, work, and try to sleep. Gums are SORE!!!

Mark really loves me now. He kept sitting with me in the chair last night and noticed tenderly how fragile and small my forearms and wrists are. He trimmed my nails. He holds me and cares for me. Part of the miracle.

April 26th

Okay, new mode, or should I say old mode. Almost exactly half-way through radiation and yesterday's blood test revealed very low white cell count. God, I was stunned but my white cells have always been sensitive to treatment. My gums are so sore it is excruciating. Still have PMS but no bleeding. Losing it emotionally. Lost three pounds. Can't eat much due to sore mouth. Should go back to more isolation and less exposure while count is so low. God, I'm going crazy here.

April 30th

Things continue to be difficult. Had absolutely no infection fighting white cells in my blood work so they would not even treat me. Instead I started the injections again to help me build new white cells. Again, the megadose. I've had to curtail the workouts and look like the POW thing. My radiation field is sore, itchy and tight.

The Mayo television show aired Saturday and was really good. Michael's photos looked fabulous. I didn't, but look better now, I think. Still have serious PMS stuff going on with no bleeding. Seems to be escalating so, soon. I hope.

Two of my employees (now former employees) told a large client that my company was on the verge of bankruptcy and that I was desperately ill and couldn't run it anymore. Then they promptly tried to steal the client. So I had to write one of my famous letters to the client explaining the truth, revealing more than I wanted to make the case.

Maybe I pulled this white blood cell number to get a break from constant treatment and to give me an excuse to back off from the company. Better get to where I don't need one.

Making plans for wearing my own hair soon. Mark and I are happy. My gums aren't sore anymore. And Butterfly Bear is taking good care of me. I'm okay.

CHAPTER SEVENTY-NINE

Dear Mom,

I can't say that I agree with your remark that God hasn't been able to answer your prayers to have peace in this family. God will not do that work for us. Instead we must look deep inside ourselves for that, which I have been doing for the past seven months. The answers come from within and God will support you while you do this work. I believe that the light we all seek in our lives is attained through the truth. No matter how painful. God will not only forgive you if necessary but will help you deal with the pain of knowing. I have also learned that it is not the duration of your life that matters. What matters is how we live in the time we do have, how we do right by others and by ourselves, and how we understand and nurture the power of love in our lives. And, unlike your remark that we have wasted so much time, I feel exactly the opposite. This is the first time in a long time that I feel that I don't waste a single moment of my precious life. I no longer pursue things that are never going to resolve themselves in my lifetime. Instead I concentrate on the positive, joyful things about myself and my family and my work and my recovery. If you will truly do what is right for yourself in honesty and truth, then everything has a way of taking care of itself. I hope you will discover this same freedom and joy in your own life. I do not believe that God will hand us peace on a silver platter. That is not how He works in my experience. He will simply give you the strength to make peace on your own.

May 4th

Okay, the shots and I made lots of white cells so I resumed treatment. Only fourteen to go. Mark and I went swimsuit shopping, a potentially very depressing deal. We got a good one though and my friend Jill will sew a special pocket into it so I can wear my breast. I'm still struggling to persevere to the end of this. Condo awaits me but I'm so deeply attached to Mark right now that I can't bear to think of being separated so long. He loves me, protects me, cares for my radiation burns, rubs my butt til I get to sleep at night and has become the ultimate partner. I love him and am in love with him. I'm free.

May 9th

Last night, I woke up around 130 am feeling strange and uncomfortable, very unsettled which is not that unusual for me these days. I began to cry and Mark tried to help but he was so tired. So I got up and went downstairs to get a cold drink of water, it being so warm in the house. I noticed all the lights were still on and the TV was going which is pretty common that time of night because Andrew is such a night owl. But Andrew was nowhere to be found. I began calling his name and no answer. Then I heard the front door open. It was indeed Andrew having gotten the flashlight from the car. He had this wonderful and mischievous look on his face, the same one he used to have when he was seven years old. He announced that there was one hell of a catfight going on outside and he was going to find them and watch it. Then he took off into the backyard with the flashlight in search of the action. I don't know what it was about that but it just made me so happy to see him so full of curiosity, energy and childishness. So I went back to bed feeling a bit better and got back to sleep. He was still sleeping when I left to be radiated so I haven't heard about the details of the catfight. A delicious treat for later, I suppose.

I have been having such a bad few days (longer actually) that I found myself slipping into some bad and very old patterns. The urge, on occasion, was to pick up the phone and call James but I am proud to say that I never did. In fact, I didn't even have to work that hard to avoid it, which was encouraging. But, damn it, he called me this morning, after weeks of no contact. Sometimes it is like he is inside my head and knows when I am the most vulnerable. I took the call and handled it decently. Always testing myself.

Only eleven more treatments to go. Almost in single digits. I'm trying to hang. God, I'm trying.

May 11th

My friend in Connecticut is running in the Race for the Cure for me today. It's very hot and I'm very sluggish. White cells hanging on but think they are dropping. Test again in a few days. I have those dark circles under my eyes. I've gone back to my Walkman for relaxation. (Jewel makes me cry.) Tomorrow is Mother's Day. I'm happy inside so I don't need the trappings. Had a really wonderful massage. Cosmic bliss.

May 14th

MEMO to Staff:

Beginning yesterday, May 13th, I wear my own hair. Okay, so there's not much of it but it's mine. Please don't look at me and feel sorry for what you think I may have lost, including a lot of long hair. Instead look at me and see what I have gained. When my doctor at the Mayo Clinic was discussing the option of a transplant with me many months ago, he said we would perform it in February and by May my entire life would blossom, just like the spring season. I watched the leaves of the beautiful, old Dutch Elm tree in my front yard fall off last autumn about the same time my own hair let loose. And now we are both covered with new growth. This is a sign of life and hope. Please share that with me when you see it, no regrets. Besides, if you think it's too punk for you, there are a lot of other management companies out there. (Don't you dare. . .don't even think about it!)

May 16th

Oh, we're turning the corner here. Today was my last day of all four views of radiation. Last five treatments are simply scar boosts. Those women techs are simply angels, that's all. The doctor asked about my breathing (fine), and any swelling (none). The nurse said my hair was darling, laid perfectly on my head. Everyone says I have a beautifully shaped head (maybe I do) and my new eyelashes are so thick. I feel free as a bird and am already in the finished radiation state of mind. Everything on the upswing. I feel life deep inside my bone marrow.

May 18th

I found the courage after my treatment the other day to venture into the chemotherapy unit. Up until now I haven't even been willing to go in there to pick up a prescription because of the intense nausea and misery I feel just having to walk in there. But I felt strong and wanted to see my favorite nurse who was the only one who could find my poor beat up veins, who understood that I would prefer not to live with a catheter any longer than I absolutely had to. I wanted her to see me feeling strong and well. It must be hard on them to administer chemo every day. Such a miserable thing. Anyway, she was there and we had an emotional talk and I got to see the others, too. The woman who dug out my bone marrow and bone sample and the one who installed my catheter the day I went into the hospital. It was simply great. I will miss them all.

I wear my own hair everywhere now. To say it is short is something of an understatement but it is mine and it is firmly attached. It is very dark brown. I noticed this morning that it is just getting long enough to start to curl up on the ends a little so I am hoping it will be curly. It is such an incredible relief to have my head free from a scarf. Sometimes it feels so light that it might fly right off.

I am almost at the beach. Thirteen more days.

May 22nd

Eve of my final day of treatment. I feel strong and healthy. Very emotional. Went to mass at 630 am. I cried through the whole thing. Felt God all over the sky after on the way to the clinic. Took a thank you card to the techs and they were glowing today. I don't know how not to be a patient anymore. Pete finished school today. We had dinner and he sweetly offered to take me to my last treatment tomorrow. But I must go alone. I'll be crying some. I haven't been sleeping so great. So much going on inside. I just don't even know what else to say. I'm alive. I'm healed. I'm happy. I have hair.
        I DID IT!!!!!!!!!!!!!!

May 26th

And so life is sneaking back to a more normal feeling without the preoccupation of treatment and its effects. But I am so much lighter, clearer and luminescent. Things are simpler, less complicated. I'm robust, Mark says. I've got a big week to get ready for the beach. I love Mark from way down. It all seems so easy and right now. From the right place.

May 30th

Dear Dr. John,
It is early morning (Day +97) and I am the only one in my office so far. Yesterday this place was lively, busy, and bustling with hard working folks. I spent the whole day here, visiting with my employees and hearing about their daily challenges, their accomplishments and disappointments, producing a lot of work myself, chatting with clients on the phone, watching the pride on the face of my top manager when I told him he was now a vice president. These are the wonderful people who kept my company running and growing while I was busy with your staff during the past eight months.

Tomorrow I am throwing a party in my own honor, having completed my treatment, and taking the whole office bowling for the afternoon. They deserve it, and so do I.

After I got home, I went to the gym, rode the bike for fifteen minutes and lifted weights for another half hour. Felt great. Why, you are wondering, am I telling you all this? Each of these simple daily tasks are so exciting and rewarding to me these days. I just love waking up and having this day, working with people I respect, enjoying my family, feeling the hair on my head, and the vitality in my body. I just find myself smiling all of the time. And, actually, when I think of it, you smiled most of the way through this thing. Or, at the very least, you always had that twinkle in your eye.

I am certain that all of your patients do not respond to the cancer experience the way that I have. But it is very important to me that you understand how your skill, talent, and commitment to the healing process led the way for me to see this as an opportunity to not just be cured, but to heal my life in its entirety. In this modern world of HMO's, uncaring physicians (such as the one who announced to me that I had cancer while I was on an operating table, wide awake, with a sheet over my face), and controlling health insurance firms, you are what I think of as an old-fashioned doctor. You took care of me, whatever it took. And a wonderful job you have done.

Now that you have given me my life back, I'll take it from here. How can I ever thank you?

CHAPTER EIGHTY

June 12th

Been a while, I know, but it was intense and busy trying to get ready to leave for so long. Mark drove me here to the beach and stayed a few days. I cried when he left. Because I guess no one needs to care for me now. Here I am in my own place alone and away from Mayo. Time to be well now.

Pete has been here last few days and it was very fun. We're so alike. I cried when he left.

I've missed writing but I'm so well. I'm too busy living.

June 15th , 3:45 am

Dear Dad,
I tried to do the Hallmark card/gift thing for Father's Day but it just wasn't happening. So I thought I would speak to you from my heart. After all, being a father is not just about getting attention over a year. It is a responsibility to do right by your kids.

Most of the problems we face as a family are because you don't wish to face your problems. This is not hard to understand, as serious as they are. While it would be beneficial for you to look at things honestly, my main concern is the real benefit it would provide to Kathy.

Ideally, Kathy should rebuild her life on her own, separate and apart from you. But the long-term abuse has had the effect of damaging her backbone, one vertebra at a time, and now she can't even stand up straight. Her back is broken. She shared with me that on this last visit, she asked you to seek counseling with her so that you could experience some relief from your "nightmares" in this late stage of your life. While it is so like her to put your needs first, as she was taught, I believe what she is really saying is it is she who needs relief from her own "nightmare." She's asking for your help. For you to deny it is a continuation of the abuse by once again making your needs superior to hers.

I know it would not be easy for you to help her in this way. It would require you to open your heart and give up the control, which has been the cornerstone of all of our lives for so long.

You asked me once, right before my transplant, if all of this had been some kind of religious or spiritual revelation to me. I was pretty preoccupied with what I was facing at that time, but now God's hand in all of this is crystal clear. It was He who understood everything inside me and created the opportunity for me to heal my disease as well as my life. And He knows the truth about what is inside of you as well. He will not do the work for you but He will love you and protect you and reward you for doing it yourself. I believe He is waiting for you to find the courage. And you will feel his approval and it will feel better than anything you have ever felt in your life. And it will assure you a place when this life is over.

On this Father's Day, I take care to acknowledge that you taught me to value and respect my intelligence and to believe that I could do or be anything I wanted. This has served me very well and I appreciate it.

Now it is time for you to use your own superior intelligence, add to it the big heart I know you have, and begin to help heal this family's wounds. Take responsibility and learn through professional help how to unburden Kathy and Mom from this terrible weight you have placed on them. Although I need nothing from you anymore, I choose to continue to believe in your ability to accomplish this. And I believe God will let you live long enough to do it. It will be the hardest work you have ever done, but the rewards will be greater than you are able to imagine. It will be scarier than flying fighters in combat and the risk to you may feel just as great. But, as a father, you could give no greater gift. And that is what I think you should be thinking about on Father's Day.

Love,

Trish

June 25th

I know I'm not keeping up. June has been a revelation in #508. Times with Mark are wonderful, full of love and joy and peace. My routine includes lots of working out, beach walking, weights, and beach laying. Had a magnificent trip back home on the seventh to give the keynote speech to the wonderful folks who regularly donate platelets to those of us who really need them. It went great and was quite a day. Not a dry eye in the house when I told my story, they say.

Michael visited for a few days and it was very difficult, as I knew it would be. Mark graciously allowed him to stay with me due to my assurances that it would be proper in every way and I really wanted to try to do it well. Didn't sleep much because it was such a strain. I have moved past Michael's favorite place, where I "put myself in his hands" (literally) so he can take care of me. I am well now and we have to find a new place together, more appropriate. He didn't handle that too well. It became so miserable that I delivered him to his sister's house which was his next stop and took a plane home for a few days. I'm just now getting back to myself here at the beach and he is coming over tomorrow to take some recovery photographs.

Dear Mark,

At this moment, I'm missing you terribly. It's you I want to be planning dinner out with and I can hardly bear going to our place with someone else. I'm so homesick for you. You were right about

Michael's visit. Too many hours. I've done a lot of listening, in fact, it might be in the category of constant chatter. That's exhausting for me so I've tried to keep a little independence. Put my earphones on at the beach so I could have a little space. Right now he's decided to walk downtown so I'm getting a little break. Because I've created this distance between us, the photos are not going great. We're working at it and hopefully it will keep getting better but he's having trouble focusing (no pun intended). This has really been a good and necessary experience for me. It has allowed me to get free of just one more thing and I recognize my response to the situation as being healthy and sound and appropriate. I had some fears coming in that have been totally eliminated. He has commented several times on the incredible change in me. How happy I am, how peaceful, and how transformed. I just keep passing tests.

Mostly I just wanted to tell you how much I love you and miss you and how happy you make me. Our last visit here was so wonderful for me. Especially the day you arrived. I felt so completely loved by you. Even when we're not together, I feel all curled up inside you. And I like it there very much. Think I'll just stay if it's okay with you. Thinking of you constantly. I am sitting in your beach chair and have been wearing your clothes.

Love,
Patricia

Had a great nap today when I returned from the airport and then watched an old Mario Lanza movie in bed. At the end, when he was singing, I had a beautiful vision out the window with moving clouds and a strange warm energy. I'm surrounded by grace and beaming inside. I've fallen in love with my husband. I'm well.

July 17th

Both boys came to visit at the beach and we celebrated Andrew's birthday. Then we drove home where we will stay for two weeks until it is time to go back to the beach for our last two weeks in August. Feel just like me. My body is big and strong. Gained five pounds at the beach which scared me to death but hope it's mostly muscle.

August 1st

Well, my two weeks at home are over and I'm on a very crowded plane back to the beach.

The two weeks have not gone well at all. Way too many hours and way too much stress at the company. Shouldn't even be leaving now but no way I can stay. I have serious doubts as to whether I can continue to live in the desert, work at this company under these circumstances and stay well. Mark seems to be slipping back to old angry ways. Kids get on our nerves. He is really feeling the stress, which is partially created by my heavy stress at work. I don't feel any of the precious love I felt during my treatment. Well, sometimes. But still got the old "you gotta carry us" feeling. Go to work, referee between angry dad and kids, messy house. Stress, stress.

And then there was my visit to Mayo. Hormone test shows that my ovaries are on vacation, which I knew already. Doesn't seem to be a problem for me, no real bad symptoms. Feels very natural not to have cycles. I love it, in fact. The doctor wants me to take tamoxifen. I don't. He says I have run the marathon and am now entering the stadium for the final lap and I should be careful not to stop until I cross the finish line.

He sent me a follow-up letter continuing to advocate for it along with my file notes regarding my history and current medical status. I always feel doomed and cry when I read those. My history is so serious — all the centimeters in my tumor and bad nodes and all. Am I going to be okay? How much do I have to do with it? What is my life about now? I wonder.

I miss the loving friendship I used to have with Michael. Because everything was so different on our recent visit, we didn't cope very well and have been struggling together ever since. I miss him.

Well, my head is spinning and there are many paths to explore yet. The healing path is the one I must find. No matter what. Perhaps dramatic change is in order.

But no tamoxifen. Can't be on drugs for five years.

August 10th

Dear Michael,
A few days ago, I felt the wind actually blowing my hair for the first time. It was thrilling for me.

You know by now that the two weeks I spent at home working were very rough. I was extremely disappointed that I allowed things to get so far off track but learned a great deal from it. There is still so much work for me to do. It is a daily job and lifelong in nature, I presume. Nothing for me will ever be the same, which is a good thing. Pete wisely advised me not to expect everything to fall into place so soon, that it will take time and will be an ongoing process. And he knows I will find my way. He is right.

August 15th

My last beautiful evening in my beloved Coronado. Sitting in my chair at the window watching the sun go down. I love every moment of every day here and always know, if all else fails, I can exist here. I've been alone since Tuesday when Mark left and have enjoyed this time so much. So I bring my recovery period to a glorious close.

Part Three

EVERYTHING SINCE

THE FACE OF RECOVERY

A short and wonderful nine months after my release from the hospital, a new year dawned, my first as a well woman. We visited my parents on Christmas Eve, reluctantly. My father had a new video camera, and as was his routine, he set it up on a tripod in the corner of the room and kept it running. It was a very difficult evening for us, and being there felt uncomfortable and disturbing. The next day my mother called to say that she had watched the tape and was concerned as to my appearance and demeanor. I was surprised that my feelings would be something she could actually see.

January 9th

Dear Mom,

While I realize that our presence at your home on Christmas Eve meets a very important need that you have, as usual, it was difficult and emotionally painful for us. Peter was particularly emotional this year, in tears on the way home. It is difficult for him to understand what is going on in this family. He understands the issues and the facts, but your role in all of it is not clear to him. He doesn't know where you stand, how you justify all of it in your own mind. He expressed a sincere need to meet with you so that you could explain it to him. You see, he has lived with not only my own pain and disappointment, but he has been consistently exposed to Kathy's challenges and seen them also through the eyes of her kids. Andrew said what may have been the only thing that could possibly have alleviated the guilt and shame I feel for having subjected my own family to so much trauma. He said that we should be grateful that our own little family was so strong and unified that we could go through these things, talk them out, and they only made us closer and better. We all talked things over with Pete and decided that maybe in the future, Christmas Eve wasn't the time to be forced to face all of the difficulties that a visit to your home brings up for us.

My first instinct in receiving your note was to immediately answer, trying one more time to explain everything to you so that you would understand, forgetting how many times I have tried that and how much I have believed in my ability to "fix" everything. I nearly spent an entire adult lifetime trying to accomplish this. Thank God cancer straightened all that out for me. It is still hard for me not to think of this as the biggest failure of my life. Not being able to heal the family after I had the audacity to bring out the truth. I still believe that the truth sets you free. I guess I didn't figure that you would not see it that way. So I am not going to try one more time to explain everything to you. That would be a step backwards for me. I am working full time on letting go of my need to do that.

Instead let me say that it is hard for me to think of you as my mother anymore because the mother I knew growing up knew me so well. She was sensitive to my feelings and really knew what kind of a person I was, what was important to me. Yet after all of the efforts I have made, the energy I have expended, you and Dad still refuse to acknowledge that my life has been more influenced by Dad's sexual illness than any other influence. All of my adult decisions were based on that influence. It almost destroyed me and my beautiful family. My disease and my treatment, in particular my transplant, saved my life. It finally belongs to me.

More importantly, I have been deeply traumatized and disturbed by the immeasurable pain I have witnessed in my sister's life. While

I have done everything humanly possible to understand and forgive, the pain and grief never subside. The books I read repeatedly stress that victims do not need the validation of the abuser or spouse of the abuser to get well. You almost never get it anyway. No point in relying on it. So Kathy and I try to help each other understand how this could have happened, how to resist the tremendous pressure you both continue to put on us to meet your very powerful needs, and how to live healthy and productive lives. Sometimes we just try to figure out how to have a conversation that is not about this. We are so worn out, so hurt and so damaged. It is one hell of a big job to try to recover from all of that. I will never give up trying. Never. I will win that battle, am actually winning it every single day. But neither you nor Dad have helped me. Instead all I hear is how much you need me to be close to you, to come back to you. My version of parenting involves more emphasis on the needs of the child. But in our family, Dad's needs came first always, and now yours are very overwhelming as well. We need some time and space to tend to our own.

Despite how terribly painful it can be, I am always grateful when Dad blurts out his theories and philosophies on the abuse. That continues to reinforce to me that he is still very disturbed and has made no progress in understanding his own problems. His recent comments included that it was "human nature" to act as he did, and besides it was so subtle that it is still hard for him to believe that it could cause this much damage. After careful examination, it would be impossible to get past that and have a happy and satisfying social relationship with this man.

As for you, all I know is that when we have contact, I am constantly reminded of the pain and frustration of this situation because nothing is resolved. There is no understanding between us. And it hurts so damned bad. In my perception, this kind of stress is the only thing in my life that has the ability to promote the growth of cancer cells. Even if that isn't true, if I assign it that power, it becomes true. I cannot feel right about myself if I overlook the atrocity that was committed in this family and try to "socialize" past it. Dad has already stated that he "chooses not to" acknowledge what happened. I doubt the two of you can truly look at it and survive. But we all make our choices and live with them.

So this year, out of respect for myself and my own family, I need a year off. No birthdays, no holidays, no pressure. Maybe time will heal some of the wounds for which I can find no other cure.

One year off turned into another and another.

As I continued to maintain my good health and keep my distance from my parents, abuse issues intensified. My sister tried to make it on her own and experienced ongoing financial problems, often asking our parents for assistance. She wrote to them in June.

June 28th

Dear Mom and Dad,

Yesterday, Mom, when I called collect from a pay phone in tears, you didn't even wait to find out why I was so upset, whether it was a cash flow problem again or if maybe I might be in some other kind of trouble. You interrupted me, as usual, and stated you "don't have any money."

Of course I understand that you are both tired of having to deal with me and all my problems. Thankfully you have Trish, the good one, and your grandchildren.

Regardless of the words themselves, neither of you seem to speak to me with love and caring in your voices, or in your demeanor. I don't believe you even know how to love me except by material gifts of clothes and the like, which are always appreciated, but they don't mean love. Neither of you believes in me or has confidence in me, never have, and probably never will.

I wonder why you should love me anyway, or why anyone should love me. I don't even love or like myself. Though plans are not fully settled in my mind just yet, I will be leaving soon and probably won't see either of you again. Everything is too painful and unresolved and apparently never will be resolved. It's the only way I can think of to salvage a semblance of endurable life for myself.

As far as you two having loaned or provided thousands of dollars for me during the last several years, I'm sorry it was necessary. Given your lifestyle, it is difficult to even believe your response to me that you "have no money." I hope you both continue to enjoy your spotless beautiful home and its lovely furnishings on the golf course, your golf outings and other pleasure trips, your shopping sprees and salon treatments, your new and reliable vehicles, your dinners out with friends, summers in San Diego and the like.

I feel that you both robbed me of my childhood and any self-esteem I may have developed if I had been raised and loved in a normal, healthy parental way. This lack of self-esteem is almost certainly irreversible. Neither of you even believe things I tell you, like my eight years of serious, focused consistent therapy, and why I needed it. You both regularly say I lie about these things.

Frankly, I feel you both should be offering to provide me with regular financial assistance as one way you should be making amends and caring for me. . .because of the way you both damaged and hurt me so badly—the horrible ongoing result of sexual incestuous abuse, committed and permitted by you both for years and years—and for the emotional trauma this abuse has evoked, affecting virtually every aspect of my behavior from early childhood until this very day. I feel I deserve and am entitled to be compensated by you both in many ways including with financial assistance. I can scarcely go a week without sorrowful crying for what I've lost, never had, and cannot find. I can barely work to support myself, cook to feed myself, or bother with my appearance. If both of you were only able to face the honest truth. . .

During my month long stay in rehabilitation three years ago, I was not diagnosed as an alcoholic or as a drug or substance abuser. I willingly share my diagnosis from one of the finest teams of professional experts in the world. I share this with you both in hopes to open your eyes and break through your very strong denial.

My three part diagnosis after 30 days of intense treatment and evaluation states:

1. Patient is a victim of unusually long-term continuous incestuous abuse

2. Patient suffers severe Post Traumatic Stress Disorder as result of this long-term abuse

3. Patient abuses alcohol as one method of avoiding the incestuous issues

I finally received validation! Something you two have never been able to give me, and that I need.

Otherwise I am only fully validated by my sister. She was there, she knows and understands. Yet she herself has never received any validation from either of you for the serious damage to her own psyche—by being exposed constantly to a home life obsessed with unnatural, unhealthy sex and sexual overtones as the constant main theme of existence. At least I validate her feelings, and she mine. This validation of each other is so overwhelming, it is the only real bond between us and it dominates all other attempts at a normal sisterly relationship.

Many people in recent years have paid dearly for sexual, incestuous and emotional abuses against their children and other people's children. We read and hear constantly now about sexually abusive incidents in the news, in the courts, in true story movies and books, often concerning high profile people, more with each passing day.

I notice often that many of these offenders committed sexual and other abuses which were far less severe and shorter in duration than what I have experienced and suffered since at least age five under your roof, "our home," for so many years—where I was supposed to feel and be safe with you both, my parents. This continued until the very day of my wedding.

I am 47 years old now, and virtually dysfunctional in so many ways. The incestuous abuses have rendered me so emotionally impaired, sometimes I feel beyond even the chance to be emotionally healthy or semi-normal, ever. Although this impairment has been a real deterrent all my life, it is seriously prevalent now, an unwelcome but ever-intruding part of my daily life. It has affected my ability to support myself, to own a safe vehicle, and to keep my modest home as my only "safe place" over the last six years.

The most debilitating years have been since early 1989, when vivid dreams triggered horrid explicit memories. The dreams and emergency sessions with psychiatrists, psychologists, and specialty therapists forced specific memories from my subconscious, gradually and in horrific detail. I wrote down the sordid details of many specific incestuous incidents under the guidance of two very helpful women therapists for four years. I relived those episodes and the more I wrote and discussed them privately with my therapists, the more I tended to recall other incidents in painful detail. Don't worry, Dad, it was very useful to me to either tear my explicit writings to shreds, or burn them in the therapist's office, once I had derived whatever relief I could by recalling, writing and discussing them in confidence. None of these writings were saved.

You two were supposed to be my "Mommy and Daddy," to love Patti and me, to take care of us, and provide for us as babies, young children, teenagers and into adulthood. You were supposed to provide a safe home and nourishment, security, encouragement and support. You were supposed to provide the kind of healthy parental love that was not supposed to include sex with me, regular incestuous behavior with me, Dad.

I don't know whether I will "make it" or if I really care anyway. Fortunately, I am not and have never been suicidal. It's not in my nature. But neither of you seems to understand or acknowledge your roles in my dysfunction and you feel I try to take advantage of you by requesting financial assistance. I am only trying so hard to continue this long-term uphill trek to emotional and mental health.

I've done my best. I've failed. I'm trying to survive. I need help.

How could you. How could you. You ruined me. You ruined me.

I am dirty and useless and cannot function. You ruined me. I am not good.

How could you. How could you. You ruined me forever. I am dirty and useless.

I will never be good or well. I never had a chance. There is no me. You ruined me.

How could you.

Kathy

July 9th

I've always had big wave dreams, terrifying visions of being overwhelmed by huge walls of water. After my recent conversations with Kathy and my father, I felt hideous, invisible, sick. Twenty-four hours of emotional chaos.

My new big wave dream: In the middle of a flat, pure crystal white desert, wandering (frolicking) in the sun. Sense of something big coming toward me, blocking the sun. See the blue wave coming. No way to escape. Prepare to try not to drown. This time the water is turquoise blue and clear with pockets of air so I can stay under and breathe until it passes. It's safe. It's even illuminating. It's peaceful and calm.

My friend from Australia came to visit and gave a presentation at my office. It was alarmingly crude for which I apologized to my employees. He was still angry at me for not spending "personal" time with him in Hawaii at the last professional conference, still smarting over our as yet unrealized affair. He knew my story from having spent time with me while in Baltimore just after my surgery. At lunch I told him how I felt the abuse had cost me the freedom to have certain experiences with men, how my sexuality erupted long after I married and had made a full commitment to my husband. How, I asked, did it feel to meet someone and act on the urge to explore those feelings. He waxed poetic on the women he had known but said it often was messy and unpleasant after. Then, with tears in his eyes, he said to me, "The things you feel you were robbed of are not precious. . . I don't even remember their names. . .I don't have anything of value. . . what you have is really important." I knew how hard it was to admit his own emptiness in order to validate my hard earned choices.

September 5th

Dear Michael,

Thanks for the chat last evening. I know there is not much you can really say but just listening is worth so much.

Having a real struggle with the full and final realization that today I have to turn in my beautiful car. Silly, you say, all this over a car when I have such a terrific replacement already. Obviously, this is not about the car even though it has been a wonderful and deeply pleasurable experience to have it.

Instead what I keep visualizing is getting in that car right after being told I had cancer, being told I would have my right breast and forty lymph nodes removed, coming home after surgery, going to the ungodly chemotherapy treatments in the car and feeling protected on the truly sickening ride home, arriving at the blood bank in it to have my stem cells extracted and leaving so weak I could hardly put one foot in front of the other, sliding into the seat that was set just for me and relaxing into the luxury and the beautiful sound. Being picked up in that car when I was released from the hospital after the transplant, mask on my face. Sliding the moon roof open often because without my long hair blowing all over, I could feel the air on my head. Trekking out to the Mayo Clinic day after day for six weeks for radiation treatments, feeling so sleepy right after that I could hardly stay awake to drive home. Being unbelievably protected at all times from the horrible things I was facing, in that car.

This morning I got up to wash the car in order to have it looking great when I turn it in. Pete was leaving for school and stopped to talk with me. We sat on the wall, looking at the car, remarking how pretty it was. He asked me how I was going to turn it in. I said I had no idea. He put his arm around me and said we should realize that this was my recovery car, shielding me from everything until I could get well. Now that I was well, it was time to step back into life in a car full of life that I could drive and experience. He reminded me what vitality and energy was in the new car, just like me now. He said it was right to retire my car for a job well done. Maybe even it would do the same for someone else. It would not be appropriate, he said, to hang on to those feelings. I must move on to life. Straight ahead. Don't look back. We agreed that we would go on a joyride in the nasty black flesheater (new car) this weekend. To celebrate life. He gave me a hug and had to leave for school. (Hard to miss a car too much when you have a kid like that.)

So I will take this step. Mourn for the loss of such a wonderful partnership, me and my car. But relish the future, now that I seem to have one. Still hurts. I'm not that tough, you know. Only when absolutely necessary.

September 20th

I go to Mayo. Have half a mammogram, a chest x-ray, and a blood test. Everything looks good, he says. Bone enzymes slightly elevated, high normal, but often the case in active people like me. I'm okay, he says. I'm okay. A cure.

I go to see a movie, A Thousand Acres, by myself. I knew abuse was the theme and was deeply proud that, without feeling shaken to the core, I endured the scene where the two sisters admitted and discussed their mutual incestuous abuse for the first time. Then breast cancer claimed the angry one, the one who had to tell. That was much harder. I wondered how many of those who see this depressing film will understand the connection between the abuse and her disease. How many will care? The reviewer said the movie deteriorated when the abuse theme surfaced. Yes, things do seem to deteriorate when the abuse theme surfaces!

And so my hair curls. And my body changes. I don't feel hurt or angry anymore. Just sad. I can let things go that don't deserve to hang around. I feel heavier, inside myself, conscious of almost of every breath I take, grateful for it, in charge of it. Nothing taken for granted. I love my husband for who he is and for loving me when I was so unlovable, for agreeing that reconstruction was not worth considering because I was so fine just the way I was, and for acknowledging life's journey and believing in my story. For knowing that I have to tell the story.

October 19th

I thought the story had come to an end, a happy ending. Literally since the beginning of my treatment I had experienced complete success. Always overachieving, the best they had ever seen at this, the fastest they had ever witnessed at that, and the incredible blessing of having been released from the constant emotional trauma of my former life. Healthy and strong, happy and secure. I knew why I had created my disease and knew that I had relied on faith and determination to put it down. So now it was down. Wasn't it?

I was originally scheduled to have my first major follow-up around Thanksgiving of last year, which included the dreaded bone and organ scans. As Thanksgiving approached, I couldn't go through with it. The timing seemed all wrong and I wasn't ready. Dr. John was very comfortable with the delay that I requested agreeing that February, exactly one year from my transplant, was appropriate. I struggled through the ordeal of tests and exams, skittish and unsettled at the very thought of it. I waited five days to get the results, but everything was fine and I saved the voicemail for months so I could listen to it over and over.

The next six month visit occurred in September and I had the strong feeling going in that this time things would not be so "pat" although I did not have a sense of a bad result. The results came back looking good with the exception of one of those innocuous looking asterisks by the alkaline phosphatas reading. He said it could be high due to exercise. I had worked out the night before the test and the morning of. Dr. John teased me for being nervous about seeing him. I was working out fanatically so I chose to accept that explanation and basically disregard the "mild elevation." My obligatory follow-up letter from Dr. John stated that he was planning to run the breakdown of the "alk phos" to determine if the elevation was in the liver, intestines, or bones. It was in the bones. The bone number is high. A high number of bone isoenzymes. Then it was him asking for a retest. Still high. Then it was him saying we could schedule a bone scan if I wanted to be "reassured" because he was quite certain it would confirm healthy bones. Instead I opted for another blood test. Same high reading. Not skyrocketing, but consistently high. We talked, me and Dr. John, acknowledging that it could be "bone involvement" from the disease, but not likely. We agreed to do nothing for now and retest in a month after I have traveled to New York for a week with Andrew. He says he is not worried and that it is a prudent decision.

All of the important people in my life consistently reassured me that I did not have bone cancer and I believed it with my heart and soul. But, oh, the fear. It works on you, gets inside of you and takes up residence, no matter how tiny the space. Dr. John sent me a fax which read "per favore, bellissima donna, non si alarma!!!!" I didn't have to know Italian to understand its meaning. He knew how worried I was. Mark's response was to draw a big heart with a tiny figure in the center with very curly hair and a big smile. Next to the heart is written, "This is my heart and you in its very center very well protected. I guess that makes you the heart of my heart. Safe and sound and beautiful." Five years ago it would have been impossible for me to feel safe and sound and beautiful and it would also have been impossible for my husband to tell me that I should. That simple picture hangs next to Dr. John's Italian fax. No woman should be lucky enough to have two such men in her life.

But that is the exterior story, the outside of the story. Inside things went all wrong, or all right in retrospect. The safety and security I had allowed myself to believe in so completely since the transplant seemed to disappear and suddenly I could only picture the horrible "what if" syndrome. Would I submit to chemo again? Wasn't breast cancer metastasis incurable? What if the transplant didn't work? That wouldn't fit with any part of my philosophy of this disease experience. I revisited every sick feeling, every intense fear I had lived through on a regular basis when I was being treated. It was such a shock. I was confused, feeling vulnerable to the disease again, knowing how dangerous that was. Crying, feeling the intense awareness of every moment of my life in the context that it felt very precious again. But there lay the clue. Somewhere along the line, I had lost sight of the preciousness of it all. I had overworked, showed myself tremendous disrespect, and generally disregarded everything my disease had taught me. I knew it was going badly, but I couldn't find my way out. Thank God I did not return to my old abuse oriented feelings of low self-esteem accompanied by the desire to indulge in old behavior addictions. Instead I was depressed and felt thick. Never light, never fresh, with no air getting through. Mark remained firm and stubbornly connected to his belief that I was well, stating that this "little hitch" was God's message to me that my transformation must be permanent and that I was losing touch with that. Time to get back on track. But for a while, I simply could not be consoled. Emotionally panicked, drained and beat.

Then I found some of the old skills, decided not to go back to victim status, and began taking charge of the situation, which gave me almost immediate physical relief. I met with my top people at the company, after investigating two serious purchase offers, and gave them the opportunity to run things first to see how well we could do. I would limit my involvement to two days a week and other isolated duties. They would step up like they did when I was in treatment. I began doing more things around the house and working out on a more relaxed schedule. I returned to the idea that I was healed and brought it to every moment of my life. Confidence. Andrew was an enormous inspiration when he validated my decision to wait another month, giving me a wonderful talk about living my life and not becoming a slave to tests. He shuddered to think what his own blood tests may look like. He even said that when we first told him that I had cancer, he was worried about the toll that treatment would take on me, but never, never worried about the outcome. He said it was one of those feelings that came from deep inside that clearly said I would survive this and it was so powerful that he never believed otherwise. Not for a moment. And he was sure it was not denial. Just complete faith. I am still riding on that conversation because I believe him.

So I am back to living "in the moment." Old cliché that may be. Mark has been out of town for several days and it has given me a wonderful opportunity to spend time alone, talk to my kids, and think about everything. I feel refreshed and reassured and, once again, grateful for the opportunity to clean up the mess that I had made in the past few months. Just keep doing it til I get it right for good.

December 1st

Ten days ago, my blood test was repeated. For some reason, they sent me to the chemo unit to have it drawn instead of the lab. It was not an easy thing to set foot in that door where I had to endure those treatments. Still makes me nauseous. It took three nurses to get blood from my tired, scarred veins. As I was leaving, I stopped to chat with a woman having chemo, bald, and tired looking. I showed her my curly hair and my fit body and told her that I had not long ago been in her chair. Literally. She thought my case was much worse than hers and considered herself fortunate that she did not require a transplant. She said she was sure that the reason I was sent to chemo that morning was so that she could meet me. She felt much better.

This time the bone isoenzymes decreased. Dr. John left me a voice mail message saying "things are looking down." They didn't decrease by very much but if the high reading was caused by disease in the bone, it would never go down, he said. Having just received the wonderful news about my bones, which appear to be active and happy, it was easy to really get into the spirit of Thanksgiving. We had a quiet dinner at home, just the four of us. On Friday evening, Mark took me to an outdoor Sarah McLachlan concert. Her music was my constant companion during the transplant. When she sang out those same songs into the cold night air under the stars, I cried like a baby, glad that I could do so. Mark drew me in close, understanding everything.

On Sunday, Peter and I played golf. On the way home, he was remarking how he would like to get the Christmas lights up on the house early this year. When we arrived home, we found that Mark had spent the day doing just that and they were twinkling in the desert dusk. We were delighted, as he knew we would be. We lit the first fire of the season in the fireplace, drank hot chocolate, and watched a sweet (okay, Mark called it saccharine) holiday TV movie together with the dogs at our feet. We commented on what a stereotype it all was and how wonderful.

And so my very first full year of recovery came to a close.

DRAGONFLIES

It is impossible to put into a timeline the moment that I first felt the presence of the dragonflies. Serious illness, particularly when laced with strong symbolic belief, opens the heart and soul in a way that is unimaginable. Exorcising the darkest forces inside leaves a light space that can be filled with new energy and power. I think it began when I saw a dainty, dangly pair of earrings in the shape of dragonflies in a store. I was drawn to them and spent a long time gazing at them, even walked away and left the store, but turned around and went back to purchase them. I couldn't explain why.

Gradually I became aware of a community of dragonflies that inhabited my body and soul, protective and inspiring. The queen was in my head, a blue dragonfly that filled my thought center. She was powerful but kind. Her presence filled me with peace but occasionally she would activate her wings at a speed that provided fresh, cleansing air throughout my body, like a high powered spiritual fan. I noticed she did this when I was feeling clogged up emotionally. I called her Willow.

She was in charge of the Black Guard, the regiment of small, feisty dragonflies in goggles that patrolled my core, protecting my organs. They zoomed around in menacing death squads, seeking cancer cells, obliterating them if found. They reminded me of the old Mighty Mouse cartoon with the familiar *Here I come to save the day* slogan.

My long bones were inhabited by the Golden Corps de Ballet. On one side were the mature dragonfly ballerinas, always working out at the barre, always in perfect unison, with high arches and strong lean muscles, dressed in point shoes and golden tutus. On the other side, the baby corps, dressed identically to their older counterparts, trying hard to discipline themselves for barre work but mostly dissolving into giggles and often falling in a dragonfly heap to take an immediate nap, wings up. The little ones grew into more serious dancers as time passed, traded their soft ballet shoes for golden point shoes and their pigtails for buns, but did not lose their joy and exuberance.

I spent time with a counselor to help me fashion the healthy, new life I had worked so hard to earn. She was part gypsy, part psychic, part earth mother and part therapist though properly credentialed. The first time we met, I was wearing the dragonfly earrings that had first attracted me in the store. She saw them and smiled, stating that she had seen me in her early morning meditation in a forest, surrounded by dragonflies. She was most pleased that I was already aware of their presence.

I now live on a lake and have the great pleasure of coexisting with the dragonflies who are attracted to the water as I am. They fill me with great joy, constantly reminding me of the beauty and fragility of life. I could not have asked for more brilliant healing partners.

Recently, I was sitting on a plane, the window seat, waiting to take off after a visit to California to meet with my literary agent. Now that the book was close to being finished, I was conflicted as to whether it was appropriate to open up my life in such an intimate way by publishing the book. What would be the consequences to my family, to others who may recognize their part in the story without yet having spoken about it openly to their own families, or to me personally. Surely I would be criticized, doubted, and scrutinized. Was I up to that? Would it be worth it? Would my story have value to anyone besides me? Gazing out to the tarmac, a large but ordinary dragonfly flew around my window. She wasn't beautiful, just brown and sturdy, darting around taking care of business. It was the sign I was looking for.

JAMES

I was instantly "cured" of my addiction to James the moment I was told I had cancer. He was wrapped up tight in my tumor and once he lived in there, he didn't have to live in my heart and mind anymore. I no longer wrote about him, not one time. My body engaged immediately in the fight for survival and renewal and no longer functioned as a receptacle for sexually soaked feelings and desires.

He became so foreign to me, almost like a dream, that I can barely remember who we used to be together. At some point, I informed him that I was very ill and a long period of time passed before we spoke again. I never stopped to think what that must have been like for him. I couldn't afford to.

As I began to experience the love and care of so many people, the space inside of me that previously required James' attention filled up with healthy emotion, peace and contentment. Gradually I developed a fear of running into him, assigning him the power of cancer itself, like exposing myself to the disease again. And I wasn't yet sure that I was well enough to withstand that exposure. So I avoided contact with him.

As time passed, I began to realize that I did not want to live in fear of him and his influence on me, that he was not cancer, and that no one had the power to make me sick again.

I talked with Mark about it one night while sitting at a bar enjoying an evening out. I asked him how he would feel if I saw James, for no other reason than to establish for myself that he had no influence over me, a test that I thought I was ready for. He agreed but I could see the concern on his face. It didn't dawn on me at the time that his concern was first and foremost for my own welfare for which he was rightly concerned, but also for his own feelings. I was so involved in accomplishing this goal of proving that I had overcome James' long term control over me that I failed to remind myself that Mark had read my journal and knew about every moment I had spent with James, everything we had done together, and all the feelings that went along with that. By understanding that it was necessary for me to confront this head on, and agreeing to it, he once again proved what a brilliant and unselfish mentor he was.

I have no specific memory of that first meeting or of hardly any of the occasional friendly meetings that followed. Therein lies the proof that they weren't memorable in any way, the proof I was longing for. He hadn't changed but was very curious about my own experience. It took him a long while to find the nerve to even hint at the notion that we weren't finished yet and it was time to rekindle the old flame, so to speak.

I had given a keynote speech at a major breast cancer event about my remarkable recovery. While I didn't specifically mention sexual abuse as the root of my disease, I did refer to a traumatic and painful event, being somewhere I shouldn't have been, doing something I really didn't want to be doing, that had triggered my tumor and created such a powerful opportunity for healing. The presentation was so well received that a benefactor of the program commissioned a documentary about my story for use in their patient and family support groups. I delivered a copy to James after it was completed and asked him to watch it so he could better understand what happened to me, not knowing if he would make the connection as to his part in that traumatic moment.

A short time later, he called saying he had watched the film. Knowing full well that he would most likely refuse to emotionally attach to any part of it, I was stunned when he said quietly and with great anguish that it made him feel "so guilty." Immediately it was clear that he completely understood, despite the fact that my film reference to our last devastating encounter was very vague. The way he acknowledged his part in my story at that moment was a profound experience for me, a kind of validation that to this day I have still not received from my father. I knew that this would allow us to stay friends, something I wanted very much, for I still believed that James was sent to me for a perfect purpose to assist with the difficult exploration of my past on my way to the future.

After that, I felt comfortable seeing him from time to time for lunch and occasionally chatting on the phone. We knew when it was time to touch base if it had been too long; we spoke about family and work and retirement and how very long we had known each other. He always made it a point to say how much he respected me and everything I had accomplished and always told me he loved me. I was so proud of preserving this friendship and considered it a positive cornerstone of my new life.

He gradually became comfortable teasing me about how long he had been waiting to have his way with me, more than thirty years, and I enjoyed it. Not once did I ever consider seeing him for that purpose or take it seriously. Not once.

We planned to get together for lunch and he asked me to pick him up. He always enjoyed my cars, partly because I enjoyed them so much, and loved to be driven rather than drive himself. After a forgettable meal, I pulled up to the curb to drop him off near his office, anxious to get on with my afternoon. He didn't get out of the car right away and continued to sit in the seat next to me and talk with no particular purpose and I recognized the way he used to behave when he didn't want to leave me. So I politely listened to him babble on and finally, when he did not get the response he was hoping for, he reluctantly got out of the car. I laughed to myself at how annoyed I was and how ten years ago, I would have been thrilled to have that effect on him and would have hung on to every extra moment as he struggled to say goodbye and watch me drive away. Off I went to the grocery store, pushing the cart down the aisle picking up things for dinner, when my cell phone rang. It was James, who didn't even identify himself, knowing he didn't have to, in his hushed secret voice telling me in detail what he really wanted to be doing with me in that car, his words laced with the old urgency and need that I hadn't felt or even thought of in such a long time. It meant nothing to me. I felt sorry for him.

Last Christmas, we spoke on the phone just before the holiday. He opened up to me about how his recent retirement had isolated him from the environment in which he had always expressed and acted on his powerful needs and now his life was centered around family including his grandchildren whom he adored. But he struggled with his ongoing need for intimacy and he felt so lonely despite being surrounded by people he loved very much. I knew he was telling me because I would understand exactly what he meant. And I did. He acknowledged how much healthier his life was since he had stopped engaging in his old behaviors and it saddened him to think of those years filled with meaningless encounters that actually left him more lonely and isolated. But for him, the intimacy he craved was realized physically, sexually. I suggested that there were healthier, more appropriate ways to create the intimacy and connection he was seeking. We said goodbye but only a few moments later I called him back and left a message to say that after the holidays, we would get together and I would help him, as a friend, explore new ways to deal with those feelings of loneliness and isolation.

Soon after the holiday season ended, he contacted me asking to get together right away. Still completely oblivious to what was going on, I agreed. When I drove up, the waitress stepped out of the restaurant to greet me at the side door and take me to where he was seated. That was my first clue. He had lost that casual, comfortable, friendly demeanor I was now used to and he was anxious and agitated. He wanted to skip the chit chat and move right to how specifically I was going to assist him with his feelings. Of course by then I understood that he had taken my comments to mean that we were finally going to consummate our relationship and enjoy the intimacy he had always longed for with me, the perfect way to fill the emptiness inside of him. I quickly explained that I had not meant that at all, that I was responding as a friend to share the many lessons I had learned through my own transformational experience. He vehemently argued that he was certain I really did mean that I was ready to be with him, that he had saved my voicemail and listened to it over and over again. He was not pleased at all when I did not succumb to his argument, obviously having completely talked himself into believing that our moment had finally arrived. He did that thing he used to do and shut down emotionally, like punishment, paid the bill, and skipped the usual warm good bye, his face dark and twisted. I watched him drive away, briefly recognizing that feeling of being left behind when he did not get what he wanted. Only this time it did not have the desired effect. I felt relief, amazed at what his behavior looked like now that I no longer engaged in it with him. And great compassion for his continuing struggle, one that I no longer felt. A short time later, and despite his abrupt unfriendly departure, I received a call from him with details of how much pleasure he was going to give me when we finally succumbed to each other. And still I felt nothing.

I avoided contact with him for a good long while after that, finally having to admit to myself that he was most likely beyond change. We still chat from time to time and he always asks if we can meet but I avoid that, making excuses about how busy I am, seeing so little point in it, and knowing that he will be unsatisfied with less than something I will never give.

I didn't tell him when I began writing a book about my life in which he would play more than a supporting role. But as soon as I got deep into the writing, to the period in which James was the centerpiece of my deeply disturbed world, he called, his radar obviously still intact. I didn't want to take the call, but because I sensed a little fear in having contact with him at such a vulnerable moment, having been immersed in my detailed James sex journal for days, I answered. I listened to him talk to me, subtly reminded him that I had written everything down a long time ago, and hung up.

MICHAEL

Even though Michael and I became close during the tumultuous years of my abuse awakening, he was not part of the problem. He was part of the solution. I always knew that we would never be together and in some ways, that is what allowed our relationship to stay so isolated and pure. We lived far apart so rarely got to see each other and the friendship had to be crafted through efforts made long distance. It developed during the days of hand written letters sent in the US Mail and Michael saved the dozens I sent to him over the years and later returned them, knowing how much they would mean to me, how much insight they would offer into my ongoing search for self. Many of them appear in this work.

He had an ability to understand me and my feelings, to know everything without having to be told. But it was never intrusive or aggressive, always gentle and subtle. As the years passed, our ability to communicate without phone calls or letters or other normal methods became frighteningly real. He had confidence in his intuitive powers and accepted them from the beginning. I discovered mine over a much longer period of time but once I did, the channels between us were wide open and we were a perfect match.

Periodically, his presence was so strong inside of me that I could barely breathe. While it was fascinating and exciting, it could also be overwhelming and disturbing, even scary. The extraordinary trust I had in him, which had never been violated even in a small way, allowed me to continue to explore our connection freely. During the most intense periods, I would finally have to ask him to leave me alone on an energetic level so that I could get some rest and go about my daily life. And he would oblige, pulling back to give me a break.

I pestered him to explain this talent we shared so I could understand it better but he refused. He said it could not be discussed in that literal way and it simply was what it was, not to be tampered with or overanalyzed, not a "parlor trick." When I got sick, it had lifesaving value. When I got well, it was somewhat more difficult to manage.

Of course I remembered the times we had spent together and the strong connection we shared. But his respect for me and my family as well as his complete understanding of my abuse-related issues kept us from exploring that connection and I relied on him for that. It was nothing like my out of control tainted attraction to James and Michael made sure that my feelings for him never got mixed up with that kind of trauma.

So I kept a special place for him, and him alone, inside of me. It took up a lot of space and was always active, vibrant and loving. I considered it separate from all other parts of my life and did not feel that it prevented me from being fully present in that life. In fact, I believed that it enhanced my life in many ways. It helped me realize myself apart from my many responsibilities and commitments. It was private and safe and I did not feel guilty about it.

It is true that there was a deep ache to fully explore the remarkable connection we had and that was particularly hard to keep under control. There were times when he was with me in a way that seemed more powerful than anything that could occur in person. I allowed myself to imagine what it would be like if we just had one week, or one day together in a place and time that held no negative consequences. It was, of course, impossible and there was no way that either of us would risk my recovery and hard fought wellness to go down that road. So I worked hard to accept it for the great gift it was, as it was, and tried to be satisfied with that.

Early one morning I received an e-mail from him at my office sent from the museum in Washington DC where he worked. It was complete gibberish and made no sense with uncharacteristic misspellings and unrecognizable words. I instantly knew that something terrible was happening to him and got on the phone to try to locate him or one of his co-workers. He was having a stroke. Luckily it was relatively mild and after a short stay in the hospital, he came home and then returned to work. It was difficult not to go there to be with him and it reminded me of how he must have felt when I was having my transplant. He had short-term memory issues, was constantly fatigued, and could no longer handle the enormous stress of his job with his usual skill. He became frail emotionally and physically, and withdrawn. His work overwhelmed him, his personal life overwhelmed him and his usual juggling skills didn't seem to be working. He even said that he had finally faced that he would never be with me and that I was out of his league and always had been. Saying such a thing was completely out of character for him.

Our relationship began to change as his life became more difficult and stressful. We had less communication and he didn't treat me with the enormous care I was used to. He was not receptive to my attempts to help him deal with his problems, and increasingly behaved as if I were demanding too much of him. It became clear that he was tossing me in with his list of responsibilities, which was offensive and hurtful. So I decided, for the first time since I was fourteen years old, that our relationship was not healthy for me and I asked him to give me some time off. He seemed shocked by my request but, as I knew he would, he honored it.

During that time, I went through the difficult emotional process of taking back that part of myself that had always been given to him through our incredible connection. It was the hardest thing I had asked of myself since I recovered from cancer and started my new life. I didn't want to give him up, to surrender that space inside that belonged to him, and us. But almost as a premonition, I knew it was work that had to be done. I took long walks and cried a lot of tears. I admitted my hurt feelings and began to get a glimpse of how liberating this work would be. Once I had accomplished my goal, I was able to feel appropriate loving friendship for him and resume our communication at no personal expense. Mostly I listened to him express his growing concerns over his life which he was now willing to confide in me. I worried about his health and state of mind, but realized that only he could decide when and if it was time to make changes and I was able to let go of our conversations emotionally after they took place.

I saw him briefly in November of 2007 when I was in Washington in my role as President of Operation Freedom Bird. For many years I had accompanied 50 Vietnam combat veterans to the Wall on a healing journey over Veteran's Day. It was the program's 20th anniversary and Michael came down at my request to take photographs of the official ceremony at the memorial to be used for my video. I was shocked at his appearance. It was a sunny beautiful day and most of us were in shirtsleeves or light jackets. But Michael was bundled up in layers with a scarf around his neck. He seemed fragile, pale and much older. He also seemed to lack his usual confidence in his ability to take photographs. I held onto his arm as we walked together as we had done so many times before in that beautiful place. I knew he was not well. And I was very worried.

The emotional work I had done during our time apart had served our relationship well. We enjoyed regular chats on the phone but they had a different tone to them, not as weighted, more friendly in the traditional way. After the holidays, he set out on a long trip with a show from his museum that was traveling to San Francisco on loan to a venue there. The owner of the artwork featured in the show had made it a condition of the loan that Michael was to be in charge and must accompany the exhibit in every phase of transport. So he had to ride in the big, climate controlled truck all the way across country with the artwork and then once the show closed, do the same to deliver the work back to Chicago. He seemed to enjoy his time in San Francisco while they packed up the show and prepared to head East, enjoying some free time exploring and photographing various California landscapes.

While on the ride home, he called to say they were going through a beautiful snow storm in Wyoming and he was getting some wonderful images. I missed that call and still have his excited message that started with "Hey, sweetheart." His voice was full of his usual enthusiasm for nature and his intuitive ability to document it. That very day I was grocery shopping at the neighborhood Whole Foods, pushing my cart, when I stopped abruptly, suddenly and completely flooded by Michael's presence. I hadn't felt that in many years and rarely ever as strong as on that day in the market. It made me gasp, took my breath away, and I stood still for a few moments until I could regain my composure. He hung around after that for most the day, his presence lingering.

The next day, after arriving in Chicago, he had promised the drivers that he would babysit the truck while they enjoyed the Patriots playoff game at the hotel. It was frigid cold and Michael took his laptop to the truck with him to work on the Wyoming photos and talk to me on the phone. We had a wonderful conversation. I reminded him what a powerful person he was, still reeling from the incident in Whole Foods. He spoke of retirement plans in the next three years or so and his second career as a private consultant that was already taking shape. He said he was feeling pretty well, feeling good about his health.

Early the next morning, his sister called to tell me that he had taken a fall on the ice going into the hotel lounge and apparently suffered a massive stroke. He was in the hospital and it was life threatening this time. She was going to get there as soon as she could. Her visit turned into six weeks as she sat by his bedside until he regained consciousness and gradually improved enough to go home with her to Texas for extended therapy and transitional care. She had seen his brain scan and described the damage as the size of a kidney all along the base of his brain, ear to ear. The doctor talked a lot about how lucky he was to be alive, saying it was unclear how much cognitive function he would regain. He was able to walk but had lost the use of his left arm and hand, a struggle that still exists today. He suffered virtually no memory loss but his speech was thick and slurred although it continued to improve.

Michael remembers everything about our past together and says that my presence was strong and vivid during the days he was unconscious. I am not surprised as I felt that I was spending every moment there with him even though I didn't travel to Chicago. I called to report a powerful dream I had about him and he already knew it, having had a similar experience the same evening with me.

I have learned a lot about strokes and those victimized by stroke in the past nine months. I traveled to Washington DC to accompany him to a meeting with a labor lawyer I arranged.

We had a lovely visit in the city, enjoying museums, our favorite restaurants, and long talks. He wasn't the same, not at all, and had trouble connecting emotionally to me. He intellectually knew that we were close, but he couldn't quite feel it in the same way. He also had difficulty preparing for the meeting with the attorney, finding it hard to get the materials organized. He was very tired after our first day and much less functional the second day.

I have struggled to cope with what happened to Michael, certainly for his sake and the great loss he has suffered. It is not clear whether he will be able to return to work or follow through with his plan to offer private consulting services. He has trouble dressing himself in the morning and hates the winter cold, which requires him to wear long sleeves, long pants, belts and coats which are harder to manage. He has a puppy, Eva, and they are very close, spending all their time together. They take long walks and she sleeps with him. I call her my "competition" because they are inseparable but he says that I have no competition. Never will, he says.

As for me, I am completely grief stricken and cannot yet process what has happened. I miss him, which is an odd feeling, because he is still there. I am grateful for so many things. It has been amazing to have him in my life all these years as such a wonderful, talented, gifted friend who contributed so much to my own recovery. My house and office are filled with his sophisticated artwork, paintings and photographs. He has taught me so much about unconditional love for its own sake. And he has always made me feel whole and loved and beautiful. I grew to rediscover myself under his tender care. We are now redefining our relationship but it is still strong and vibrant.

I recently went to see a psychic intuitive. You are instructed to leave a voice mail before you arrive and from that sound she prepares note cards with various names on them relevant to your life story. Michael's came up right away in my session. She said that rarely, if ever, had she been witness to such a strong connection between two people as I obviously had with this man. She also said that his greatest work as an artist would be post-stroke and it would also be his most commercially successful. He has yet to pick up a paintbrush but I am hopeful that he will.

MOTHER AND FATHER

Several years ago, after long-term estrangement from my parents had been well established, I wrote to them anticipating their use of a strategy destined to fail. At the time, both parents were healthy and active filling their retirement years with golf, travel, and social events. My letter outlined my suspicion that they would hold out until one of them became ill or incapacitated at which time they would expect me to come dutifully to the bedside in question and absolve them of all their sins. I made it clear that the longer the estrangement continued, the less likely that was to happen and that the natural course of life and death would not influence my position. I was interested in healing, truth and the hard work of reconciliation. There would be no instant fix in this matter. Despite my best efforts, the strategy was put into place. There was no reaching out, no response at all to my letter. And time passed with only the occasional outburst of anger and disbelief that I would dare cause this nonsense to continue year after year.

My father's health began to decline and my mother looked carefully at each step to find something that rose to the medical standard of "estranged daughter comes home to reconcile with ailing father on deathbed." We could always tell when the standard had not been reached because no specifics were given. I was still naively struggling with why there wasn't an "abusive father has revelation that causes him to beg forgiveness of daughter before he dies" moment in the works.

The search for a diagnosis began, seeking that magic medical word that would be powerful enough to reunite the family, my cancer being the sought after gold standard. But there were just vague speculative answers from doctors as in "might be this, might be that." But whatever it was, it seemed clear that he would continue to lose his faculties and sink into a world of his own, filled with hallucinations and delusions. I was told that some days were better than others, with the better days downplayed and seemingly apologized for while the bad days were highlighted over and over again. My mother wrote to say that one day she found him leaning forward in his chair while watching television, with tears running down his face, murmuring my name. I was told how rare it was for him to shed tears and this was surely an omen that he must see me before his imminent death. Subsequent visits by my sons produced stories of various justifications on the part of my parents as to what kind of person I could possibly be that could create this unjust punishment of them along with what a cold, unfeeling, uncaring person I had become. I was briefed on how pathetic my father had become and what a sweet "impotent" old man he was. It was my mother who was terrorizing the family now. My parents were still an inseparable team, each sticking with the other no matter what the consequences. Losing the love and affection of a child seemed to be considered acceptable collateral damage.

Despite my decision made years before that his looming death would not bring me back, the reality was difficult. I knew I wasn't the terrible person they made me out to be and was used to being served up on the silver platter in that way. And I knew they had not taken even one tiny step towards acknowledgement or acceptance of their own culpability, still telling family in South Carolina where I had loved visiting as a child, that they had no idea what made their daughter stay away from them. The silver platter became a familiar place, just like home. Even after more than twelve years of splendid recovery, my father's illness and decline nudged me towards collection of memories, digging deeper than I had before. It was during his decline that I began to write about my life on the silver platter, the art of being served up over and over again.

As the pressure continues to mount, I make the decision to stay away each and every day. My son, Peter, armed with his intuitive gift, reports that my father negotiates with him for my quick and easy return. I will come over one evening, he will say he did some things wrong, I will say I did some things wrong, we will have dinner, and that will be it, will be enough. No plea to produce me so he can put things right, ask forgiveness for his grievous wrongdoing. Instead he just needs that one visit from me to grant him absolution. I have believed for some time that it will be hard for him to let go, to die, still estranged from me. How would it look, after all, if the entire family were left to forever wonder what terrible thing could have kept his daughter away while he was dying. No, he much prefers that they say that his daughter finally came to her senses at the very end and by doing so, proved that it was she who had the issues, not him. Once again, I would take up residence on the silver platter. And ride it all the way to the funeral and into eternity.

I still believe that I am part of God's plan to encourage both parents to find the courage to face their own lives and by so doing, provide the healing and comfort that my sister and I have so longed for, and that they so desperately need. If I were to validate their lack of courage, all hope would be lost. Yes, I believe that God is validating my decision. And as my friend Kathy says, the world does not support such decisions as refusing to minister to your dying father who is suffering just down the road. You must be brave to be so bold.

And yet I remember the letter I wrote years ago to my parents urging them to support my sister's therapist as he recommended that she avoid contact with them during therapy. My father's response was that if she continued to do that, she was "dead" to them. But when I was facing death by high-risk cancer and bone marrow transplant, my father did not come to me to make it right, even after I told my parents that my cancer was abuse and my transplant a method to clean out the toxic trauma. No, he was completely willing to let me die without the benefit of the truth to comfort and validate.

My legacy, the power of my story, is my willingness to stand up in the face of enormous pressure for what I believe is right, just and fair. Not only for me, but for all of us who have ever been controlled and manipulated, used and abused. For the God given right to say no. The world may not support that decision, but God does. Let that be enough for each of us. Please God, let that be enough.

GINA ROSE

Regina Rose loves to tell the story that she flew into my transplant room in a basket fueled by helium balloons. As part of a gift basket sent by a client, I guess you could say that she's right. Regina is a storyteller and admittedly takes liberties with the facts on occasion. We indulge her that. Besides, we can almost always tell when she is fibbing. She has a very active imagination.

Butterfly Bear and I were happy to welcome her to our room, grateful for the company. But she was quite the little snot in the beginning. In fact, we named her Regina because it was clear she thought she was the queen of everything. It took her a while to warm up to us and come down off her high horse, an expression my mother used to use with me when she thought I was getting too uppity. So me and Regina had a little something in common from the beginning. But I didn't let on.

She was absolutely oblivious to the fact that she was a teddy bear, adorable though she was. No, Regina seemed to have a distinct personality, an active presence, and an opinion on just about everything, even though she didn't speak in the beginning. I was drawn to her energy and understood her immediately. With nothing but time on our hands in the sterile room we called home, I felt my childhood imagination begin to emerge through my connection with this little bear, and suddenly my goal to recapture the innocence and joy of myself as a little girl begin to take shape.

One day, Regina found her voice. Out loud. She began speaking, we began conversing, and before I knew it, we became each other. I gave her a voice, a literal voice, different from mine. She was funny, serious, opinionated, creative, passionate and a little arrogant. She gave me a way to express the simple joy of a life that had, in part, been taken from me a long time ago. Through Regina, I was able to say whatever I wanted and see life through the filter of a child's eyes. Things I could never say as my adult self were suddenly coming right out of her mouth. The sweet side of me that I was trying to recapture was comfortable in Regina's care. She helped me express the things that I missed so much about myself, that I had locked away for safekeeping. Regina could sing and knew all the words to musicals, Barbra Streisand songs and hits of the 60's. With my help, she could kick high and do the splits and dance. What a pair we made. Butterfly thought it was hilarious and continued to try to fly all over the room and misbehave and hide from us. For this, Regina would reprimand him.

By the time I left the hospital, Regina had become a friendlier Gina Rose and we were best friends, inseparable. We saw things the same way, and validated everything for each other. It wasn't clear whether she would ever make herself known to anyone else but that would be up to her.

One night after our release from the hospital, Mark and I were lying in bed. Gina and Butterfly were hanging out with me as usual. Suddenly with no warning and out of the blue, Gina jumped on Mark's shoulder and said, "I can do the splits." He was a little taken aback, but because he is Mark, took it very seriously and responded with appropriate respect. Once he let her know that she would be taken seriously, Gina began to blossom and Mark became her new best friend. She told him everything she thought, demonstrated her diving technique including multiple somersaults and twists, and shared her dreams of being in the Olympics. She also confided in him about her broken and difficult childhood, raised by her mother, Babia, the Solar Queen, a selfish and powerful woman who did not care about her little daughter, leaving her to fend for herself. Gina and I shared a passion for children who were not properly loved and nurtured by their parents.

Gina was able to find a soft spot in my Dutch stoic husband that no one else had ever accessed. He forgave her everything, indulged her shamelessly, and immediately dropped a bad mood or sharp voice to interact with her. It was like she developed a direct line to the sweetest part of him. This was a revelation to us all, Mark included. Gina had given both of us permission to care about each other in a way that our adult sensibilities had prevented in the past. She gave me the courage to trust this most tender part of myself with Mark and in return, he shared the most vulnerable part of himself with me. How she loved being our love sponsor.

With Mark's support empowering her, Gina showed herself to Andrew and Peter who were used to their mother's slight craziness and took it with a grain of salt. One day the larger of two family dogs, Rusty, grabbed Gina in his mouth and took off running throughout the house. Rusty, being an enormously gentle animal, meant no harm and made no effort to hurt her, but Peter, with his own flair for the dramatic, chased him around and claimed Gina from what she would later say were the jaws of rape and certain death. This only contributed to her theory that men are dogs (except for Mark, of course, and now Peter).

Gina became a sports fan and fell madly in love with little Stevie Nash of the Phoenix Suns, admiring his unselfish play and commitment to teammates. Because he was shorter than the usual NBA player, she declared him a perfect boyfriend candidate and was crushed when she found out he married his longtime girlfriend and they had twins. She was a loyal and true fan of every team she adopted, even when they performed poorly. On big game days, she would sit quietly in meditation for hours, signifying for a good outcome.

In early March of 2008, Gina decided that she had a lot to say about the world and wanted to become an Internet blogger. She created Just a Bear with a Blog (jabwab.com) and began to write early each morning about whatever was on her mind, whether it be politics, the arts, or acts of kindness in a complicated world. This gave her a forum for her opinions and beliefs and storytelling. She wrote about Rusty when he died, telling about how on his last night on this earth, she begged his forgiveness for telling the story of how he almost raped her when actually she knew that he meant her no harm and was just having some fun. She wrote of the power of his forgiveness. She wrote about her search for her own birthday and the tough times as a teddy bear on a shelf in a store with hundreds of others who looked just like her and her fear that she would never have the chance to become herself. She wrote about the great hurt and disappointment in her unhappy childhood. She wrote about her boyfriend, Nicky, the former Dominican monk who was a little frumpy and quiet but fiercely loyal and who really understood her, wondering if it was enough. She wrote about how lucky humans were to be able to have so many choices every day to do simple things that she could only dream about doing. She wrote about dragonflies and hummingbirds and Zen philosophy and seeing Tom Jones in person in Las Vegas. She wrote about how one day she hoped to have her own radio show, The Regina Rose Show.

It was through this little bear alter ego that I found my own voice. The blog was an outlet of huge significance to me, allowing me to express everything that had been inside of me for so long and could find no way out. It was a way to speak to my own family and let them know certain things about me such as how much I loved them and how I saw them for who they are. It was a way to reach out to other women who were having the same struggles and who responded to Gina's openness and sweet, simple perspective on our lives. It gave me the discipline and confidence to believe that I could write this book.

When I was a child, I was fascinated by the relationship between Sherri Lewis and Lamb Chop, connecting to it in a powerful way. When Gina appeared, I remembered that feeling and knew that I could have that same opportunity with her. Our relationship is a key component of my continued healing as she helped me reclaim a part of myself that I loved and missed terribly. When we merged, Gina and I both experienced a huge boost in our self-esteem. Sometimes we look for what we want and desperately need in all the wrong places. When it's right there before our eyes.

SISTER

My sister was a willowy five seven at just under a hundred pounds when she was younger. No, it was not an eating disorder. She was just lucky, well-proportioned and slim. Shortly after I got married, I went to the East Coast to visit friends and my sister came up from her home in Montgomery, Alabama to see me. I saw her standing in front of the mirror, nude, getting ready to go out and was struck by how beautiful her body was, boyishly thin but still mature in a female way. She was radiant that day, physically perfect.

All that changed as the powerful result of sexual abuse began to take hold in our family. When the truth emerged, and Kathy's secret was no longer secret, she began to drink and eat and cry and crumble. There was a moment when one word from my father, mother, or the both of them, admitting what she had endured and offering support and validation would have saved her. But that moment never occurred and it was not enough that I was there for her, having had my own share, and knew the truth. It was our parents and them only to whom she assigned the power to fix everything. And they had no intention of doing so. They saved themselves, expecting her to take the fall for the family. And she did. And she does. Every single day to this day.

Her body began to change, under the assault of her increasingly addictive behaviors. She became alarmingly promiscuous with a serious alcohol problem. With a life spiraling out of control, and parents doing everything possible to deflect the blame away from themselves, my sister gained weight. Lots of it. Every pound she has gained is a reflection of the intense emotional pain she lives with each day. She has an exaggerated need for privacy, often dreaming that she lives in a glass house where my parents can see her at all times. She takes two glasses of water to her bedside at night so that she can choose which one she wants to sip from. She relies on various prescription drugs to keep her functional and has a doctor who sees her only for the purpose of monitoring the combination and dosage of the brightly colored pills. She hasn't worked in years and lives very modestly in a small house using the money that my parents and I send each month. Her health insurance is provided by the state. After a visit with our parents, she can sink into a deep depression, crying for days, sometimes weeks. She rarely goes out of her house.

It became increasingly difficult for me to visit with my sister in person or by phone. Her needs were emotionally overwhelming and her continuing connection to our parents had a way of making it impossible to speak about anything but our unfortunate and unresolved family secret. I felt I had done my own healing work at great personal risk to myself and was very protective about not allowing myself to slip back into the dark abyss of the family dynamics. Seeing her in such an emotionally debilitated state made it difficult not to address the abuse issues, the root cause of her dysfunction. She supported my decision to stay away from our parents, understanding that it would be risky for my health and well being to have contact with them. But she believes to this day that she and I can have a relationship separate from the parental problems. My family and I do not agree. She once told me, in an uncharacteristic moment of openness, that her therapist said that

I was the only one who was handling all of this in a healthy way. She is still deeply entrenched in her life-long training to serve the needs of my parents before her own. She sometimes stays at their home assisting with our father's physical care at great emotional expense to her.

Obviously the sexual abuse my sister endured for so many years at the hands of our father is far worse than my own. I write my story in her honor, to show my respect and care, and to acknowledge her voice, still silent.

For her I harbor the same hope that guided me through my own recovery. The hope that one day she will remember and retrieve the wonderful, bright, healthy, caring and loving woman that she is inside.

AS FOR ME

After my eight months of cancer treatment ended, I couldn't imagine electing surgery that was not lifesaving for any reason whatsoever. But Dr. John felt that I owed it to myself to visit with the plastic surgeon and discuss reconstruction. My medical team did not even consider allowing reconstruction to take place immediately following my surgery due to the high-risk nature of my diagnosis. Save my life first and then worry about the cosmetics. I reluctantly agreed to the consultation. Dr. John had arranged my appointment with the best plastics man on the Mayo staff, highly experienced with national recognition and credentials. But he had a "fellow" under his tutelage at that time and he was the first face I saw. A young, brash man, he grabbed my fat file and began to examine its contents. Knowing nothing about stem cell rescue, he took one look at my diagnosis and apparently concluded that my prognosis wasn't all that great. After a few moments of review, he looked up at me and subtly suggested that reconstruction probably wasn't for me after all. Why, I asked? He said it could be a long and difficult process and in my case, it probably wasn't worth it. You know, because I wasn't going to survive anyway so why bother. Just enjoy the time I had left and let it go. Once it dawned on me what he was really saying, my first instinct was to crawl into a hole and die, just as he was predicting. But by the time the visit was over, I somehow found the courage to confront him, in a much more emotional state than I would have liked. How dare he imply that my case was terminal? What did he know about my treatment and prognosis anyway? Luckily, I was tough enough and had enough faith and belief in myself that I would go home and after a few days of very hard work, would come to know that he was wrong and I would not allow his shocking suggestion to become a prophecy. I was determined to ensure that he never had the opportunity to say something like that to another woman again. I wrote a long, detailed letter to his superiors and received a prompt reply saying he was no longer in the Mayo program. With apologies.

I never seriously considered reconstruction anyway. There is something about my flat strong chest on one side that seemed right, like the important part of my story that it actually is. It looked like it did when I was a little girl, partly because my large port wine birthmark covers the red surgical scar making it hardly noticeable. It isn't like I lost the opportunity to wear bathing suits and low cut tops because my birthmark has always been an impediment to that. I came to believe that my father was right when he said that God gave me the birthmark for a reason. It prevented me from seeing my body as a sexual power tool. It wasn't perfect. It set me apart in my own unique way. As a woman with a story. And yes, I do believe it is God's mark on me just as Mammy said, a result of a bolt of lightning in a Southern thunderstorm.

After several years of persistently high "alk phos" levels in my bones, and absolutely no acceptable answers from Mayo as to what could be causing the only post-transplant number that was out of line, I figured it out myself. I was losing bone mass and heading straight to osteoporosis. Once my ovaries shut down as a result of high dose chemo, I went into instant menopause placing me at high risk for bone loss. A bone density test was ordered and the results confirmed my theory. To cover their astounding medical "miss," my doctors insisted that I go on a bone-building drug. Just as I had refused a long course of tamoxifen, I also refused bone-building drugs. I would figure it out on my own, I said. And I did. First my bones stopped their downhill slide and then began a gradual recovery. Having made every cell in my body, feeling an intimacy with them, I was determined not to insult them with more drugs. I would just ask. We worked it out.

The instant menopause caused almost immediate and shocking weight gain, which I had experienced in my lifetime only when pregnant. Since no member of my medical team warned me of this, I was horrified and resented the surprise. While I enjoyed life without menstrual cycles and birth control, the body changes were completely unacceptable. I made bold diet and exercise changes, worked out every day and watched what I ate. It helped but I was still unsatisfied. Finally I committed to a serious training facility and worked myself into great shape, losing five percent body fat in the first year, gaining six percent bone density and getting to know the former dancer I used to be again. I allowed myself to be completely open with the people who supported me at the facility, telling my physical and spiritual story, and in the process, added another important piece of the puzzle in reconnecting to the whole woman I wanted to be. One of the massage therapists there told me about Bikram Yoga which I now practice regularly. It adds a continuing connection to spiritual and emotional renewal while providing a workout for my organs, which they appreciate very much. It has been incredibly empowering to rebuild a body that matches the mental and emotional strength necessary to overcome not only my disease, but that which made me so ill for so long.

I had the great pleasure of running into one of my transplant nurses at the Mayo Clinic when I was in for a long-term follow-up appointment. She was delighted to see me doing so well and with a head full of curly hair. It dawned on me that once transplant patients leave the unit, those who cared for us at the most critical moment of our lives have no way of knowing what happened to us, whether we even survived. She gave me a big hug and I told her how honored I was that she remembered me. She told me that everyone remembered me. When I asked why, she said that they all knew that something was going on in my room. While they weren't sure exactly what it was, everyone wanted to be in there, to be part of whatever it was. What drew them to my room was not just the music, it was the healing that was taking place there. It was the rebirth of a life. It was hope. It was love.

Now I truly feel like myself. Yes, I have two different colored eyes. Two different colored hands and arms. A breast on one side and none on the other. A back that is half red and half white. And a brain that works a lot better on the right side than the left. Like I said, I feel just like myself.

THE LOVE OF A CHILD

When Andrew was a baby, we took him to visit Mark's parents in Iowa. I had only been there once before, a short time after we married. Considering that his mother, a smart Irish Catholic woman, did not approve of our four-year cohabitation and completely ignored our wedding day, things were not going well. I overheard her in the kitchen on our first night there bitterly complaining that I had left food on my plate. From that point on, I took small portions and small seconds. I dreaded bringing my baby to her beautiful home, still somewhat insecure as a new mother. She had put an old family crib in her room on the main level for Andrew instead of upstairs in the big dorm room where Mark and his brothers used to sleep, next to our room. I was horrified that my little boy was going to be close to her and not me in the night. Mark told me to settle down and let her have her way.

The next morning, she announced that we would be moving the crib upstairs. I was thrilled but couldn't imagine what could have caused her change of heart. She explained that when she awoke very early, Andrew was standing in his crib saying "mama." My mother-in-law couldn't bear to keep us apart after the child virtually asked to be with his mother. It was the first time that one of my sons made me feel cherished, but certainly not the last.

When Peter was less than a year old, I left him with Mark and Andrew in Colorado and went to Florida to spend a few days at the beach with my mother and sister. Unlike Andrew who was a feisty, independent baby, Peter was an intuitive, sensitive child who seemed as though he had sprung directly from my DNA. If I was too tired to get up in the night, he would mysteriously skip his feeding. If I needed a nap, he would take one, too. When I arrived home from the trip, Mark said he was asleep in his room. I tiptoed in just to lay my eyes on him. He was standing quietly in his crib in the muted afternoon light, waiting for me with a beautiful smile, dressed in a pale yellow, soft, one piece suit with snaps and feet. I reached for him and took him in my arms. It's funny how you remember such small moments. When he put his arms around my neck, I felt completely whole and completely loved.

My Oprah inspired sexual abuse awakening began shortly after that incident while we were still living in Colorado. Gradually it took over my emotional life and overwhelmed almost everything for a very long time. To this day I feel it robbed me of making a full commitment to my own family, which was the most important thing in my life. Over the years I began to believe that the abuse issues had prevented me from showing physical affection to my sons when they were growing up and that maybe I had held back too much, preventing them from feeling the enormous love I had for them. One night, well after my recovery from cancer, I took my family to dinner and delivered a prepared speech about how sorry I was that I hadn't been able to be the mother and wife I should have been due to the distractions of the terrible family secret. They assured me that I was everything they could hope for in a mom and my concerns were just silly.

We chose to be completely open with our boys about my father and what happened in my family. As they grew to be adults, I encouraged them to have their own relationship with their grandparents, urging them to base their decision on how they were treated, not how I was treated. So despite my long estrangement from my parents, my sons continued to visit them on holidays and birthdays. When my mother was critical of me or my decision to stay away, they warned her that a condition of their relationship was that they never be asked to choose sides, that their loyalty to me was absolute. Andrew once had lunch with my mother for the sole purpose of telling her that she would never win that battle, that he and his brother would always choose their mother over her. Privately, based on their own observations, they insisted that I stay away, believing it was too risky for me to ever go back into an environment that was still every bit as toxic as the one I left behind.

When the boys were growing up, my father purchased a big, clunky video camera and shot home movies that included holidays and soccer games and fun afternoons at their pool. While we were sometimes irritated at him for shooting such events, I now consider those tapes priceless. A few years ago, I asked Peter to see if he could talk my father into lending me the old VHS cartridges so that I could transfer them to mini-DV which would allow me to edit them myself. Reluctantly, he gave them up long enough for the transfer to take place. When I first saw the tapes, I was overcome by emotion. There was deep affection in the images, closeness, and so much love between me and my children. It was then that I knew for sure that even the hideous journey through sexual abuse had not taken from me the ability to love my family, to show them how much I loved them. Love is more powerful than abuse. And I am living testament to that.

How strangely beautiful that the love of my children could provide for me the validation and feeling of being cherished that I did not receive, and to this day have not received, from my parents. Because parents shape the formative years of our lives, their actions are necessarily foremost in how we come to view ourselves. And we all live with the consequences of that upbringing, good or bad. But my children have taught me that love is a perfect circle, and sometimes while we are so busy seeking what we need elsewhere, we fail to notice that those needs can be or are being met through a different kind of love. My children have been raised to value themselves and have great confidence in their own value. Their love for me is unconditional and they make it easy to accept it without question or doubt. While I was mourning the loss of my parents' failed connection to me, I became a parent myself and it was my own children that helped fill the empty space inside. The perfect circle of love.

I have learned that what my father did was wrong. He is a deeply flawed man who never found the courage to acknowledge his own problems and the enormous suffering they caused. I have learned that my mother is another of his victims, shaped and molded by him from the age of nineteen. Had she been able to stand up for me and my sister, or even believe us, the healing and validation would have been transformational for the three of us, and maybe even for my father as well. It has been hard to accept that he has chosen not to take responsibility, and as a very sick, old man, it seems clear it will never happen. It has been much harder to accept that our mother, even in the face of facts virtually admitted by our father, has chosen absolute loyalty to her husband over the silent screaming of her daughters for motherly protection, love and care.

And so we must learn to care for ourselves. Make love where there is none. Shape our own lives with the values that are important to us. Do it for ourselves and each other. And when you are lucky enough to be loved for yourself, and to love yourself and others, make sure you are fully present in that love. Don't make it less important because it is not the love of those who let you down. When a child puts their arms around your neck and holds you tight, when your husband or lover cherishes you in a healthy relationship, and when you feel the joy of loving a friend with all your heart, allow that love to exist fully inside you. If you don't feel it in your life, keep seeking it, but always remember that it can be enough just to love yourself. That is the real journey.